PRAISE FOR

Law School Confidential

"The   e many,
and   ensively.
Valua   chool. A
usefu

"This   out law
schoo

"Mille   surviving t   makes
this b

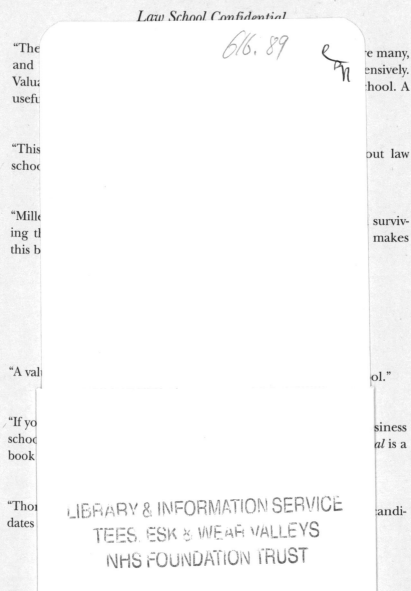

"A val   ol."

"If yo   siness
schoo   *al* is a
book

"Tho   andi-
dates

MED SCHOOL

SCHOOL

CONFIDENTIAL

ALSO BY ROBERT H. MILLER

Law School Confidential

Business School Confidential (with Katherine F. Koegler)

Campus Confidential

MED SCHOOL CONFIDENTIAL

A Complete Guide to the
Medical School Experience:
By Students, for Students

Robert H. Miller

AND

Daniel M. Bissell, M.D.

ST. MARTIN'S GRIFFIN
THOMAS DUNNE BOOKS ❧ NEW YORK

THOMAS DUNNE BOOKS.
An imprint of St. Martin's Press.

MED SCHOOL CONFIDENTIAL. Copyright © 2006 by Robert H. Miller and Daniel M. Bissell, M.D. Foreword © 2006 by Harold M. Friedman, M.D. All rights reserved. Printed in the United States of America. For information, address St. Martin's Press, 175 Fifth Avenue, New York, N.Y. 10010.

www.thomasdunnebooks.com
www.stmartins.com

Library of Congress Cataloging-in-Publication Data

Miller, Robert H. (Robert Harrax)
     Med school confidential / Robert H. Miller and Daniel M. Bissell, M.D.
         p. cm.
     ISBN-13: 978-0-312-33008-8
     ISBN-10: 0-312-33008-1
     1. Medical education—United States. 2. Medical Students—United States. 3. Medical colleges—United States. I. Bissell, Daniel M. II. Title.

R745.M612 2006
610.71'173—dc22

                                                                2006044414

CONTENTS

ACKNOWLEDGMENTS

WHILE ANY AUTHOR would love to claim the finished product as the jewel of their creation alone, the truth is that there were many important contributors to the book you now hold in your hand. First, a thank-you for the invaluable input and insights of our fantastic mentor group. Thank you Ben, Chris, Deb, Pete, Carrie, Adam, and Kate. It is your contributions that have transformed an otherwise unilateral impression of medical school into a broad and comprehensive guide to the experience. We appreciate the time, the effort, and the candor you offered, and are honored to share the authorship with such an august and talented group. Thanks also to Nancy Nelson, former Dean of Student Affairs at the University of Colorado School of Medicine, for her encouraging words, extensive contacts, and sage advice; and to Dr. Andy Perron, Program Director at the Maine Medical Center Residency in Emergency Medicine, for allowing his chief resident to write this book, and for his superb support and encouragement.

We would also like to thank the many people who contributed to *Med School Confidential* behind the scenes. First, to our terrific literary agent, Jake Elwell of Wieser & Elwell, who has stood by the Confidential series from the beginning and has helped to nurture and grow it into the well-respected, international platform it has become. Honors three times, Jake, makes you a CB Club Member. Thanks also to Tom Dunne and Pete Wolverton at St. Martin's Press for seeing the wisdom in turning the success of *Law School Confidential* into a series.

On the production side, true thanks go to John Parsley, our editor at St. Martin's Press, who inherited this project, but whose enthusiasm, responsiveness, and professionalism have kept us on track and made this book his own. John, we're truly grateful to have had the chance to work with you. Thanks also to Mark Steven Long for an exceptionally good job copyediting and fact-checking.

Finally, a thank-you to our families for unending patience and support in the face of tremendous pressures and long hours.

From Rob: To S.D., for seeing me and our family through yet another *Confidential* entry by so ably and loyally manning the rudder while I continued to insist on fiddling with the sails. Your many contributions to this book, to all of the others, and to the dreams of an aspiring author looking to make good on those dreams will never be forgotten.

From Dan: To Kim, who shouldered the burden when the teetering tower of residency, research, kids, writing, and life seemed about to topple over. As always you kept our family moving forward and filled me with inspiration to get the job done. Your contribution to the final section of the book has given a voice to the countless spouses who have also weathered the med-school experience and will be inspiration and solace to those who come behind us. Thank you, also, to my father for brandishing the red pen one more time and bringing thirty-five years of teaching experience to bear on our piece, even if it did run a bit over the five-paragraph limit. Your insights, instincts, and insistence on proper punctuation were invaluable.

FOREWORD

THE TECHNOLOGY AND organization of American medicine is evolving rapidly and it constitutes not one career path. Medicine provides options for students with diverse interests and personalities. There are some unifying themes: you need an ongoing interest in science, concern for people as individuals, high ethical standards, and a willingness to work as part of a team. These qualities must be present in any physician, whether he or she contemplates a career in primary care, a more narrowly defined clinical specialty, administration, or bench research.

Your genuine interest and enthusiasm for biological science must persist over an entire career. The advances of the year 2006 will give way to a more advanced understanding and a new vocabulary in just a few years. To maintain your accreditation, state licensure boards demand proof of continuous education efforts. Specialty certification is now limited, in most instances, to a decade before a recertification examination is required. If these challenges are odious, humanitarian motives alone will never be an adequate substitute. Very few of us are really scientifically creative, but you must be excited about the advances appearing each week in the best peer-reviewed journals. These advances must impact the care of your patients.

Science has its limits, though. If you do not see yourself as a laboratory researcher, you must not squander your college years taking highly specialized science courses you will soon forget and probably never use. You must pay more than lip service to a liberal education. Some exposure to subjects like English, economics, political science, history, a foreign language, art, and music can immeasurably enrich your life. You still must do well in the required premedical sciences:

general chemistry, organic chemistry, biochemistry, biology, and physics. Be sure to take these subjects at your home college or university or at an institution of equal academic stature, not an inferior school because you fear the grading curve on your own campus.

All physicians who care for patients must be interested in them as individuals, not bodies with a diagnosis. You must be a competent communicator. Be willing to speak but also be able to listen. You must be sensitive to cultural and educational differences that may color a patient's perception of their illness and may require you to modify your usual approach.

High ethical conduct must be engrained in your character. Advances in health care rarely seem to decrease cost. You have an obligation to try to be certain the new technology or drugs are cost-effective, not just something new with marginal benefits. Cost containment and rigid practice guidelines, when based on good clinical data, may save resources of both society and your patient. Everything you do must be tempered by the notion that your first obligation is to your patient and not to enhance your own income, the group's, or an insurance company's.

Health care has become more complex than even a few years ago. The solo practice of medicine is a distant memory for most physicians. You must be comfortable working as an important but rarely omnipotent member of a team of health-care providers, many of whom may not be addressed as doctor.

As mentioned earlier, not all physicians choose to be involved with largely full-time direct patient care. Research in an academic institution may have strong appeal either in patient-based studies of a new drug or procedure, or at a cellular level. You must always remember that your work must be directed at improving the life of your patients.

Whatever your ultimate calling in medicine, this thoughtful book will aid you in better understanding the process of medical education and help you find your way.

—*Harold M. Friedman, M.D.*
Associate Professor of Medicine (Emeritus)
Chair, Admissions Committee,
Dartmouth Medical School

PART ONE

So You Wanna Be a Doctor . . .

INTRODUCTION

Is there anyone so wise as to learn
by the experience of others?
—Voltaire

THERE IS, PERHAPS, no more outwardly appealing career than medicine. It is hard to argue with a career choice that allows you to save lives, or at least improve them, every day. Doctors are also well-compensated and enjoy job security largely unparalleled in today's society. The fact is, the world will always need doctors, and doctors still garner a level of credibility and respect in our culture that lawyers, entrepreneurs, and other highly compensated professionals have long since lost.

So what about medicine? What is it that is drawing *you* to it?

Maybe your interest has been triggered by those enduring, romantic perceptions, by a family member who is a physician, by Hollywood's depiction of doctors, or even by pages from a biology textbook. Somehow you developed the notion that a life in medicine might be just what the doctor ordered. But what would that mean? What does a physician's life look like?

How hard is it to become a doctor?

By picking up this book, you've taken a crucial first step, meaning that you're either interested enough in the idea of medicine as a career to want to explore it further, or that you've already committed to the idea and are looking for guidance and perspective. This book can help you on both fronts.

Together, in the pages of this book, we will embark on a journey of discovery through truly foreign territory. The lexicon will be, at times, arcane and tongue-twisting, the structure, hierarchy, and traditions often seemingly byzantine. Between the covers of this book, though, you will find a detailed map of the world of med school and advice from an elite group of mentors to guide you through the perils and pitfalls of the premed and med-school years. This book contains the wit and wisdom, insight and inspiration to take you from your first musings about medicine as a career through medical school and the beginning of your internship—and everything in between. By reading this book, you will gain invaluable knowledge and perspective about the process, which will enable you to approach medical school with confidence and excitement.

Let's begin!

HOW TO USE THIS BOOK

THIS BOOK BREAKS the medical education process down into its six component parts, each part representing a major step on the journey to becoming a doctor. This structure allows you to either follow the steps sequentially, if you're at the beginning of your journey, or to jump right to where you are in the process. Each section of the book contains an overview, discusses the challenges unique to that section, and offers specific guidance about how to survive and thrive in the experience and advance to the next stage of the process. In each section, your team of mentors—people who have all just been through the ups and downs of what you're about to experience—will highlight the critical aspects of the journey, steer you around the pitfalls, and help you separate what is important from what is not. Spend a moment reviewing their biographies on the next few pages. Your mentors come from diverse backgrounds and very different med-school experiences. By learning from their successes, mistakes, and misadventures, you will make important distinctions and gain insight into what matters and what doesn't.

In a moment, we'll be introducing you, the reader, to your mentoring team—the group of just-graduated med students who will guide you with their advice, wisdom, and anecdotes throughout the following pages. First, though, a bit of advice about how to get the most out of this book. It has something to offer you, whether you are a college student thinking about med school, a working person contemplating a career change, a student already in med school, or the parent/friend/significant other of a med-school student and you're just trying to understand what your loved one is going through. De-

5

termine which of the following situations is most applicable to you, and read on.

I am a college student thinking about applying to med school/I'm thinking about changing careers and applying to med school

If your med-school experience has not yet begun, you've just stumbled upon a wealth of information and resources that will make your entire experience easier, less stressful, and, we hope, more successful. We suggest that you read this book from cover to cover before you begin the application process (1) to confirm for yourself that you really *do* want to go to med school, and (2) to get a good overview of the entire experience to help inform your interviews and application essays. Once you've familiarized yourself with med-school terminology and gotten a sense of the process, you should then go back and read each of the individual chapters as they become applicable to you.

I've already been admitted to med school, and I'm nervous . . .

Yeah, well, join the crowd!

Almost everyone entering med school is nervous about it because of the mystique associated with the experience. You, however, have come to the right place at the right time. Unlike your classmates, who will fumble nervously through the first year not knowing exactly how to proceed, you will have a step-by-step proven plan—a map of the road to success drawn from the experiences of the mentoring team you're about to meet.

Take the time between now and your first day of classes to read this book cover to cover. Don't worry if you don't understand everything right away. Just familiarize yourself with its content and with some of the basic ideas and concepts it presents. Then, when med school begins, keep this book within arm's reach and let it be your guide through each month and each year of the experience, steering you safely around the pitfalls and hurdles into which your classmates will stumble. Use it to measure your progress and to keep track of where you are.

This is your book of wisdom. Let it work for you.

But I'm already in med school . . .
I wish I'd found this book sooner

Yeah, us, too. The difference between you and us, though, is that at least you can still benefit from this book. We had to learn most of this stuff the hard way!

The fact is, it's never too late to start. If you are already in the throes of med school, we still recommend reading the entire book, as there are earlier hints and suggestions on which you can still capitalize. Then simply go to the table of contents, find where you are in your med-school career, and begin in earnest. Read forward to the end of the book to get a feel for what's to come, and then concentrate on specific chapters as they become applicable to you.

If you could get help in the middle of an exam, you'd take it, right? So what makes this any different?

I'm the parent/friend/sibling/significant other
of someone going to med school

Want to give your friend or loved one the best gift you could ever give them at the times they need it most? You have it in your hands. Before you wrap it up, though, you may want to skim it yourself. In it, you'll soon discover why your med student isn't returning your phone calls, letters, or e-mails, doesn't have time to come home to visit, and is frequently tired and cranky when you call. If you are close to a med student, their experience will touch you, too—and the better your understanding of its incessant demands on time and energy, the easier it will be to accept the virtual loss of your loved one for the next eight to ten years. The impact of the stress, the schedule, the financial implications, and the emotional swings of med school is very real. As such, part seven of this book includes a chapter just for you, written by Dr. Bissell's wife, containing accumulated wisdom from family members and partners to help you see your med student through this challenging process.

Your job is to be as supportive, understanding, and forgiving as possible, and to place as few demands on your med student as you can. Reading this book will help you to understand why—and also give you some familiarity with the experience they're having.

That said, it's now time to meet the mentors who will guide you through the next four years and beyond. As you progress through this book, you'll be able to follow their course, discover and learn from their mistakes, and watch their careers develop before your eyes. You can and should model some of their actions, choices, strategies, and experiences. And you will learn from all of them. You see, at the end of our med-school careers, many of us walked away shaking our heads and muttering to ourselves, "I wish I knew then what I know now." You are in the unique position to have that wish granted.

It's time to get busy!

CAROLYN COME
Newton, Massachusetts

B.A. Cornell University
(Government)
M.D. University of Vermont Medical
School

Premed: At Cornell, as an
undergraduate

Time off between college and med
school: 2 years

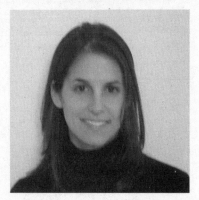

After college, I took a position as a research technician in an immunology lab at Brigham and Women's Hospital (the same lab I had worked in the summer before my senior year of college). I worked in the lab for two years. My projects involved the use of murine models to explore the relationships between T-cell-mediated immune responses and atherogenesis.

MCAT prep: Kaplan

MCAT administrations: 1

Number of med schools applied to: 20

Number of times applying to med school: 1

Residency: Internal Medicine

Both of my parents are doctors, so growing up I had a lot of exposure to both the rewarding and difficult aspects of being a physician. I was always impressed by my parents' devotion to and compassion for their patients and their patients' families. I also saw the affection and regard with which my parents were held by their patients. I think I first thought about becoming a doctor in high school because I liked science, and I thought I would enjoy doing what my parents did. At the same time, I often wondered whether I really wanted to be a doctor or whether it was the only profession I knew much about. While I took all of the requisite premedical courses in college, I chose to major in political science because I loved reading and learning about government and history. After college, I did research in a lab for two years to help me decide whether I wanted to pursue a medical education. My time in the lab increased my interest in medical science and experimentation. Pursuing a medical career offered me a wonderful opportunity to combine my interests in science and working with people.

Overall, I am very satisfied with my career in medicine. I sometimes think, when I am exhausted, that I wish I was doing something less physically and emotionally stressful. But, usually, I cannot think of anything else I would rather do.

CHRISTOPHER CREAN
Charlotte, North Carolina

B.A. Holy Cross (Chemistry)
M.D. Georgetown University Medical
School

Premed: At Holy Cross, as an
undergraduate

Time off between college and med
school: 2 years

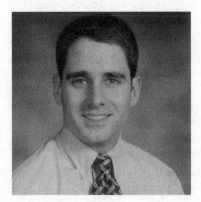

I took two years off between college and medical school. I knew I wanted to have at least one year away from the books, and I believed gaining some life experience would make me a better doctor, if not a better applicant.

The first year after school I joined a volunteer organization similar to Americorps in Portland, Oregon, working for an AIDS social service organization. It was actually a great year, and I was given a firsthand look at the AIDS epidemic. It was rewarding work, and I think it will make me a better physician down the road.

My second year, I moved to Boston to be closer to my then girlfriend, now wife. I worked at Boston Medical Center in the pediatric HIV clinical research department. My responsibilities were split between assisting in clinic and data entry. Again, it was a rewarding year, giving me another perspective on the medical field. But after about six months I knew I wanted out of the nine-to-five world and was ready to start school again.

MCAT prep: Kaplan

MCAT administrations: 2

Number of med schools applied to: 15

Number of times applying to med school: 1

Residency: Emergency Medicine

I spent some time in the hospital as a child, thankfully only for simple ailments like appendicitis and an open fracture. At the time I think I was too young to consider medicine as my future profession, but the time spent in the hospital certainly gave me some insight into one of the basic responsibilities of doctors; they help make scared, sick people better.

Studying science and mathematics had always been an enjoyable activity for me. As I got further along in my schooling and started looking for ways to become a part of the scientific community, it became obvious that I was not meant to do bench work my whole life. I enjoyed working with people too much. Teaching, at least in a classroom setting, did not seem to be for me. In the end, the more I contemplated it, the more medicine just appeared be a good fit.

I am exceptionally happy. I love what I do, I look forward to coming to work, and I enjoy the people and the patients I get to work with.

DEB FAULK
Longview, Washington

B.A. University of Denver (Biological Sciences)
M.S. University of Denver (Biology)
M.D. University of Colorado School of Medicine

Premed: At University of Denver, as an undergraduate

Time off between college and med school: 7 years

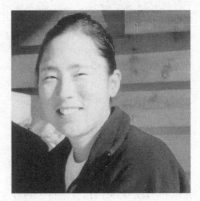

I applied straight out of college and was wait-listed at one medical school but didn't get in, so I got a master's degree in biology, and then spent four years as a laboratory technician before reapplying.

MCAT prep: reviewed on my own, using Flowers and Silver's *MCAT* prep book (Princeton Review Series), known as the Flowers book

MCAT administrations: 2

Number of med schools applied to: 5 the first time, 1 the second time

Number of times applying to med school: 2 (seven years apart)

Residency: Anesthesia

The road to medical school was a seven-year adventure for me. I actually was convinced in high school that I would be a doctor, and I applied straight out of college. The day the final rejection letter came, I had to shift gears. I decided I would go to graduate school, finish my degree in a year, and reapply for medical school. Well, one year turned into three, and in that time I realized that I was not really that upset about not getting into med school. Was that just my ego protecting itself from the reality of rejection? Maybe. But in any event, I was too tired to go through the application process again. With my master's degree in hand, I entered the world of research as a lab tech. For four years, I spun test tubes and tortured mice—but I also worked with many an M.D. I actually started to get the bug again. I mean, I realized I couldn't be a lab tech forever. I wanted to do more, but if I knew nothing else, I knew I didn't want to get a Ph.D. The whole grant-writing thing just wasn't for me. Besides, to really do research at that level, you needed to have a burning question, and I had no burning questions to answer. I did have, as anyone deciding to go into medicine has, an inflated sense of wanting to help others. Most of all, I had a mission to prevent others from experiencing the unnecessary suffering that I had gone through.

You see, in my first year of graduate school, I tore my anterior cruciate ligament in an indoor soccer accident (I am now very pro-grass, anti-turf!). Anyway, I was met in the ER by a friend who cringed along with me as the doc tested the stability of my knee, and who drove me home after being shown the X-ray revealing I had a bone chip broken off my tibia, which would take about six weeks to heal. After six weeks of dutifully keeping on the straight splint they told me to wear, I was frozen in about fifteen degrees of flexion with quadriceps that had atrophied to nothing. Besides which, my leg felt as if it was twisting off every time I turned a corner. Something was definitely not right. I went back to the doctor and saw a physician's assistant, who again tested the stability of my knee and thought it felt fine. However, with my symptoms and the mechanism of my injury, he thought it prudent for me to get an MRI. Five weeks later, the proper diagnosis was made: "See this large empty space on your MRI? That's where your ACL is supposed to be." After four weeks of waiting to see an orthopedic specialist, two months of physical therapy preop, the operation itself, and six months of physical therapy postop, I could finally bend my leg and almost walk with a normal gait again. I knew this could have been prevented, and I thought I was the person to prevent it from happening again! Med school, here I come.

I am very satisfied with my career in medicine. I am happy to report that I picked the right specialty! I really do enjoy anesthesia. It still feels like I am neglecting aspects of my life while trying to complete my residency and master all of the skills and knowledge I am supposed to master during my three years, but in terms of the specialty and practice of anesthesia I know I made the right choice. I actually had a self-affirmation of sorts this year. I had a baby in March 2004. My department was more than supportive during the pregnancy as well as afterward, while I was out on maternity leave. I was worried that like many of my friends, I would be torn when I had to go back. I was pleasantly surprised to find that while I missed my baby Jake (of course), it also felt great to be back taking care of patients and learning again.

PETER E. SEDGWICK
Holden, Massachusetts

B.A. Williams College (Geology with
concentration in Environmental Studies)
M.S. University of South Florida, Tampa
(Geology)
M.D. University of Massachusetts Medical
School

Premed: As a postbac at Harvard Extension
School

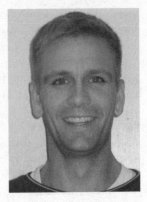

Time off between college and med school: 7 years

I spent seven years between the two, first figuring out what kind of life I
wanted as a person, then figuring out the best way of achieving that life. My
first year after school was divided between working as a boat bum in the Ba-
hamas, working on a farm in New Hampshire, and guiding kayak trips in
Baja. While the life was good, there was little I was contributing to society,
so I went on to get a master's degree studying the effect of sea level rise on
coastal erosion. Here the contribution to society was present but was too
abstract and academic for me to want to pursue long-term. Teaching high-
school-age kids for the next two years both as a prep-school teacher in the
Virgin Islands and as an outdoor trip leader in Australia, British Columbia,
and the Western United States provided an excellent outlet for my goals of
affecting positive change in the world—but looking thirty years down the
road, I knew myself well enough to know that there would not be enough
academic stimulation to stick with it. Working as an environmental activist
with low-income communities in East Oakland, California, between my
postbac and medical school cemented my commitment to social change
and reinforced for me the tremendous impact one person can have on a
community.

MCAT prep: reviewed on my own

MCAT administrations: 1

Number of med schools applied to: 9

Number of times applying to med school: 1

Residency: Family Medicine

I made the decision to go to medical school while working as a high school teacher. I loved learning wilderness medicine for my outdoor guiding work in the summers, and I was looking for a way to continue to do a career involving community service yet still have academic challenge and personal growth at the same time. I had been out of college five years—one of traveling and working odd jobs in beautiful locations, two of graduate school (master's degree in geology), and two of teaching high school. It was not until that time that I even considered the option of medicine, even though my roommates in college were predominantly premed.

I love my work but hate my job. Medicine is the most rewarding and amazing profession to enter into, with magic around you every day. There is a scintillation of life, death, fear, joy, and pure distilled emotion at every turn. You touch people at a level that no one else can really understand. You can be the best thing that ever happened to someone in their life, ever, simply by being capable at what you do and being kind at the same time. Whenever I get frustrated, I think that I could be behind a computer doing finance, or selling something to someone else, or working in middle management, and I realize what an amazing field I have chosen for my life.

The price for this, however, is high. You lose sleep, gain weight, develop sleep disorders if you are lucky and emotional disorders if you are not. You neglect your loved ones around you at times, at others you neglect those patients in your care. You battle endless bureaucracy and paperwork with little to show for it. You get abuse heaped on you at times by the people you are trying to help. I will never forget the day a senior resident said to a group of interns, "Has everyone had that moment where they have thought about driving into oncoming traffic?" Everyone had.

BEN SMITH
Middlesex, Vermont

B.A. Princeton University (English)
M.D. Columbia University Medical
School

Premed: As a postbac at the
University of Colorado, Denver

Time off between college and med
school: 5 years

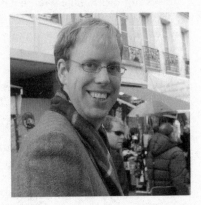

I was a newspaper reporter for about a year and a half before making the
decision to do premed classes. I loved the job for its intensity and the way
you got to learn about so many things in such a short period of time, but I
wanted to be able to offer something more concrete in return to the
people I was learning from.

MCAT prep: Princeton Review

MCAT administrations: 1

Number of med schools applied to: N/A

Number of times applying to med school: 1

Residency: Emergency Medicine

My decision to become a doctor was a very conscious one, which I made
after finishing college and doing other work for a while. I wanted a job
that gave me the opportunity to know and learn about a wide variety of
people while offering a concrete service in return. It also seemed to me
that there was a self-reliance, or autonomy, to the profession that felt attractive. None of my family was in the medical profession, so it was quite a
departure in a way.

Medicine is an incredibly exciting profession. It changes you. But I urge people to consider the time costs, too—eight to ten of the prime years of your life given to this profession, meaning you can't do other things a lot of the time. Your friends will be surfing at Laguna Beach, tailgating, and hiking to Machu Picchu while you do rectal exams on vomiting cirrhotics who never say thank you. But once in a while, you will also do something that saves someone's life or makes it better. You might deliver a baby or diagnose someone's diabetes and change their life. You will learn things about people (both in particular and in general) that few others will know. I think it's important to be clear about the trade-offs. It is a significant sacrifice to be a doctor. If you understand that and still want to do it, then it is incredibly worth it.

ADAM SPIVAK
Baltimore, Maryland

B.A. Princeton University (English Literature)
M.D. University of Maryland School of Medicine

Premed: At Princeton, as an undergraduate

Time off between college and med school: 1 year

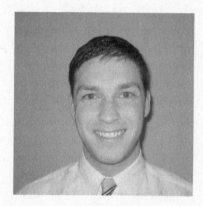

I decided during the beginning of my senior year that I was going to take one year off after college and before attending medical school. I found a nonprofit group based in Utah that ran Peace Corps–like programs in countries around the world. I ended up working for them in Bolivia, spending seven months living with the Aymara Indians.

MCAT prep: Princeton Review

MCAT administrations: 1

Number of med schools applied to: 20

Number of times applying to med school: 1

Residency: Internal Medicine/Infectious Disease

As far back as I can remember I always wanted to be a physician. My father is a practicing hematologist. He never put any pressure on me to become a doctor, but I think the example he set with his professional life had a very strong impact on me.

I am very happy with the way things are turning out. It is the best job in the world. One of my professors told us that if you are in medicine for the right reasons, you are in for the time of your life. I am looking forward to an academic career in Infectious Disease.

KATE DRUMMOND
Conway, New Hampshire

B.S. Bates College (Biology with a secondary concentration in French)
D.O. University of New England College of Osteopathic Medicine

Premed: At Bates, as an undergraduate

Time off between college and med school: 3 years

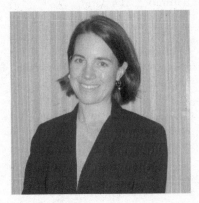

I took three years off after college. I felt that it was important for me to gain more experience, to live in the real world and save some money. I worked as an EMT paramedic for the local fire department, taught EMT classes, worked at an emergent care clinic, and was on the local ski patrol. These experiences helped me make sure that medicine was truly a lifelong career for me. I was also able to get out in the real world and away from being a full-time student. I matured as a human. I strongly recommend taking time off—it will not jeopardize your chances or choices.

MCAT prep: prepared on my own, using *A Complete Preparation for the MCAT* (Betz Publishing Co.), known as the Betz guide

MCAT administrations: 1

Number of med schools applied to: 3

Number of times applying to med school: 1

Residency: Emergency Medicine

I can't say exactly when I decided to become a doctor, though I do recall coming home from kindergarten and watching *Emergency* . . . I was fascinated by Johnny and Roy. My early inklings became more concrete in high school. I began to teach for the American Red Cross and became an EMT shortly after graduation. I began volunteering and working as an EMT immediately, and continued this through college and the three years before medical school.

After college I was working in an emergent care clinic staffed by both M.D.s and D.O.s. I found that D.O.s had a little something extra to offer to their patients—manual manipulation. I learned more about this technique and the theories behind it while working at the clinic. This provided me with the exposure that I needed to make the decision to pursue an emergency medicine career as a D.O.

Overall I am very satisfied with my career. I honestly cannot picture myself doing anything different. True, there are days when I wish I was bagging groceries and my only worry was bruising produce or breaking eggs. But then I step back and look at how far I have come and what an honor it is to play a role in very vulnerable moments of people's lives. The one downside is the litigious society that we live in. It can be challenging going to work each day knowing that a mistake can end your career. So practice wisely.

CHAPTER 1

Thinking About Med School?
Think Again . . .

Know thyself.
—SOCRATES

CHOOSING A VOCATION, particularly one like medicine, is a daunting task. Our social programming starts early in childhood, through role modeling, media portrayals, and questions like: "What do you want to be when you grow up?" Some people have an early, seemingly innately directed passion for a particular field that they pursue headlong from day one. For the rest of us, the path is more circuitous. Whatever your own course has been thus far, if you now find yourself contemplating a life in medicine, you must take the time to consider how it is that you got here.

Find a quiet place where you can be undisturbed for the next twenty minutes or so. Turn off your cell phone, your MP3 player, and anything else that can disturb you. We're about to ask you a series of very serious questions, the answers to which will reveal much about your readiness for medical school. After reading each question, write in stream of consciousness, in the space provided, everything that comes to mind. Do not organize, filter, or censor your thoughts. And don't worry about writing in the book! This book will be your tool and your guide through medical school and residency. Break it in and make it your own.

Get everything down on paper. You may be surprised at what you're about to learn.

Take a deep breath and try to relax.

Ready?

Go.

THE FOUR QUESTIONS TO ASK TO ASSESS YOUR READINESS FOR MED SCHOOL

1. How did you end up considering medical school?

_____

_____

_____

_____

_____

_____

_____

_____

2. Have you considered other career paths? Why or why not? Which other careers have you considered, and why did you abandon them?

_____

_____

_____

_____

_____

_____

_____

_____

3. What are your three primary motivations for pursuing a career in medicine?

_____

_____

_____

_____

_____

_____

_____

_____

4. What do you imagine a career in medicine would be like?

_____

_____

_____

_____

_____

_____

_____

The amazing thing you'll discover as you get deeper and deeper into a medical career is the great variety of answers to these seemingly basic questions. What is it that attracts people from all avenues of life, and all stages of life, to a field that involves such incredible sacrifice—a commitment of seven or more years of your life and an investment of hundreds of thousands of dollars? While it is impossible to catalogue all the reasons advocating for or against a career in medicine, there are some common threads that bear discussion.

THE TOP FIVE REASONS *NOT* TO GO FOR IT

The easiest place to start is with some of the common myths and misconceptions that often drive people toward a career in medicine. Go back and look at your responses to the questions above. If any of the following reasons appear in your responses, you may want to more thoroughly examine your decision to explore medicine.

My parents were physicians

Family traditions are great, but if you're contemplating med school just because someone else in your family is a doctor, think again! A career in medicine requires such deep personal commitment that the mere desire to carry on family tradition will pale in comparison. If you have physicians in your family and find yourself intrigued by their lives and careers, then by all means draw on them as resources, talk candidly with them about their experiences—and then reach your own conclusions. You're charting your own course here, though, so make choices that work for you. If you're getting pressure to pursue medicine from doctors in the family, ask them for an honest response to the question, "Would you do it all again if you knew you were going to start your career in medicine in the world as it is today?"

Remember, you're the one who will be awake all night studying. If your motivations aren't strong enough, you'll likely end up unhappy.

The money and prestige

In general, physicians are well compensated for the demanding work they do. The days of your M.D. degree being a ticket to glory as the neighborhood millionaire, however, are clearly over. As a by-product of the current health-care crisis, physician salaries have stagnated and even dropped, despite increasing pressures, increasing costs, and diminishing rewards. If you choose a career in medicine, you will definitely be able to lead a comfortable life, and you will definitely be able to pay back your loans. But if your motivation for pursuing a career in medicine has more to do with a fancy car, a low handicap, and a beach house than it does with patient care, you might want to go back to the drawing board.

I can't think of anything else to do

In deciding to go to medical school, you should be pursuing a chosen dream, not evading indecision. Pursuing a medical degree is not a casual undertaking, and anything less than your 100 percent commitment plus a complete knowledge and an understanding of your purpose for being there will likely cause you to falter somewhere along the way.

It's okay to be concerned about the decision, to ponder it heavily, and it's even completely appropriate, maybe even customary, to have some misgivings after you get started. Once medical school begins, however, indecisiveness about your overall commitment to medicine is at best disempowering and at worst crippling. As Ben notes, "The best advice I can give to someone thinking about medical school is to remember that medical training is a very intense (even brutal) eight-to-ten-year process during some of the prime years of your life. If you are excited about that, then go for it."

You must seriously evaluate your options and your intentions in advance, so that if you choose to proceed you can do so with confidence. Even more important, you can articulate to yourself a thoughtful and convincing defense of your decision to pursue a career in medicine when the going gets tough.

The adrenaline rush

The practice of medicine has been described as "hours and hours of sheer boredom punctuated by moments of sheer terror." This axiom certainly applies to medical school as well. If you have bought into Hollywood's glorification of medical practice, though, be forewarned. Clinical practice can be exciting, and, yes, on a day-to-day basis you do manage to save lives, sometimes even in dramatic ways. But most of the days of your medical career will involve caring for the three-year-old with an ear infection, a ninety-year-old from the nursing home who is weak and dizzy, and the alcoholic with poorly controlled diabetes who has just vomited on you for the third time. It's true that you will thrive on those cases that require quick, decisive action and get the adrenaline pumping, but your more gratifying work will often be the run-of-the-mill stuff that really involves you in people's lives and allows you to connect with them and make a difference. In general, those who are addicted to the adrenaline rush and focus solely on that miss not only the elegant subtlety of the profession but also ultimately wind up unhappy and unfulfilled.

I want to help people

This one probably stopped you in your tracks.

You probably thought this was the reason you should be going to medical school, right?

Well truthfully, this *is* a noble reason for pursuing medicine. You should be aware, however, that there is a yawning chasm between the sentimental image that society has of doctors providing compassionate care for all in need and the practical realities of the resource-limited, highly politicized version of medicine actually practiced today. If you have an altruistic heart and really want to make a difference, you should absolutely consider going into medicine. But be aware that defending the purity of your intent and staying true to your guiding altruism will be a constant and central challenge to you every day of your life. If you succeed, you'll not only directly serve your own patients, you will also lead by example and help change medicine for the good of all. To succeed, though, you'll need to overcome the progressive dominance of business and greed in our cumbersome and failing health-care system.

"Those who I believe make excellent physicians are those with caring, compassion, and a desire to make people's lives healthier in the true sense of the word," Pete says. "Unfortunately, these are also the people most frustrated with the limitations on how we practice medicine today and they are least likely to find satisfaction in the financial rewards and quality of life of a doctor today."

So how did you do?

This is an admittedly harsh list. Our intent here is not to dissuade you from going into medicine, but to be provocative and ensure that you consider your decision carefully. Of course, most people pursue medicine for a host of different reasons.

Now, consider our list of positive motivations below.

THE TOP FIVE REASONS TO *GO* FOR IT

I want to help people

"Wait . . . what? But you just said . . ."

That's right. This item is on both the lists of pros and cons. As discussed above, altruism is, in fact, a crucial part of the physician's character and should be a fundamental guiding principle as you enter clinical practice. At the same time, you need to be acutely aware of the contrary forces of business and profit motives that are significantly influencing the profession. Go in with your eyes open. Altruism is a powerful motivation—but your restraints on practicing it will be one of your primary frustrations and sources of dissatisfaction.

There is no doubt you will be frustrated and angered when lawyers, businesses, and governments tell you how to care for a patient and force you to leave good science, common sense, and compassion by the wayside. Nonetheless, you will also discover that every ounce of empathy and comfort you offer to your patients will be repaid one hundredfold, and that these are limitless resources that cannot be stipulated, dictated, or overruled. It is this wealth, ultimately, that will keep you returning to the bedside day after day and night after night.

I want to apply my love of science to my love of the humanities

Medicine is an elegant blend of the sciences and the humanities, of the technical and the creative. It encompasses every field of science and has ever-expanding horizons. Your interpersonal skills and so-called emotional intelligence will invariably be challenged by the diverse array of patients you treat, and you will come to know and be involved in the most intimate aspects of their lives. You will, at different times, find yourself a scientist on the frontier of knowledge, a teacher making the abstruse facts of disease and treatment clearer to the frightened patient, and even a spiritual guide helping a dying patient on his final journey. Medicine will constantly test every aspect of your intellect and personality, and it will never cease to teach you and make you grow. Who could ask for a better job than that?

I am fascinated by the human body

You'd better be!

For the rest of your working life you will be deeply embroiled in the inner workings of every aspect of this most amazing machine. Even if you are not a biologist at heart, you must have an appreciation for what our bodies achieve and the elegance with which they are constructed and operate. This respect will be a source of inspiration during the darkest hours of Anatomy or at the bedsides of your sickest patients.

I want to build on my existing experience in patient care

Perhaps the best way to clarify your intentions about medicine is to try it hands-on. If you've already done some volunteer work—as an EMT, for instance—or otherwise dabbled in the clinical setting, you have likely gained important insights into the joys and tribulations of working with patients. If you walk away from those experiences finding yourself eager to go back for more, chances are you'll be inspired in medical school.

I can't imagine doing *anything* else

Some have said that because a career in medicine requires such immense dedication, the only reason to pursue it is if you truly can't imagine doing *anything* else. We don't take the analysis that far. Suffice it to say that for some, a career in medicine has been a clear and lifelong dream. Those whose dream has also been well thought-out and scrutinized tend to do well. For others, however, the discovery is more gradual—that postcollege, nonmedical jobs just never quite satisfy or fulfill the way they think a life in medicine will. Whichever route you have taken to get here, just be certain that you have adequately scrutinized that route and properly confirmed your choice.

A REALISTIC SELF-EVALUATION FOR MED SCHOOL

If you have satisfied yourself that your motivations are proper, the next question you're probably asking yourself is, "But can I do it?"
"Am I good enough?"
"Am I smart enough?"
"Am I dedicated enough?"
These questions are all very common to prospective medical students looking up at the daunting mountain they have to climb. It's time for some more introspection . . . as the answers to these questions must come from you.

Am I smart enough?

There's no question you need to be a solid student and a clear thinker to be a good physician. Indeed, the premed process often seems less about preparing you factually and more about confirming you are an accomplished student who can manage volumes of complex material. This doesn't mean, though, that if you haven't breezed through your premed course work you won't make it in med school. We all had strengths and weaknesses and premed classes that didn't go as well as we'd hoped.

As a whole, you should be able to perform solidly in your premed classes in order to feel confident approaching medical school. Interestingly, the challenge once you're in medical school is less about the complexity of the material and much more about managing the sheer volume of it. While there will be times when your intellectual mettle is measured, more often than not it will be your organizational skills and not your brilliance that will be put to the test.

Am I disciplined enough?

Your discipline, commitment, and ability and willingness to focus on your medical studies are arguably the most important considerations in this list. Not only is medical training intense and arduous on a day-to-day basis, it's also interminable. Day after day, your self-discipline will be tested and stretched.

Can you keep up in Anatomy so that you're not overwhelmed come test time?

Can you juggle Pathophysiology, Pharmacology, and Histology tests all in the same week?

Can you remain sharp and engaged at 3 A.M., when your team is admitting your seventh patient of the night?

These challenges will tax you to your absolute limits, but getting through the experience will be one of the most rewarding things you'll ever do. Ultimately, your self-discipline will be fundamental to your career and will be a long-standing source of satisfaction that you can call upon for the rest of your life.

Do I have the perseverance?

Okay, assuming that you're smart enough and you're disciplined enough, your next concern will likely be whether you have the stamina to endure when the going gets tough.

Medical training can be a dehumanizing process. You will often feel humbled by your peers—convinced everyone in the room is smarter than you. You will frequently be taken to the depths of exhaustion and then asked to do more. After weeks of little sleep, you will be asked a difficult question by an attending physician and then humiliated in front of others for not knowing the answer. The experience can truly shake your confidence to the core. This is why you must know, with absolute clarity, why you want to become a doctor. It is this certainty that will give you the fortitude, conviction, and self-respect to persevere.

Am I too old?

The general answer to this question is no, you're never too old to consider medical school.

If you're an older or a second-career student, however, it behooves you to be realistic about where you are in life and what your expectations are. There are many doctors practicing medicine today who had a major career shift and went to medical school as late as their fifties. If you have the drive and the passion, go for it. But recognize that much about the eight-to-ten-year course of medical training is truly grueling. It means hours and hours of studying, nights up on call, and long periods away from your family and loved ones. While older students may find themselves more adept at balancing their lives and efficiently navigating the med-school waters, they will not escape the very real physical and emotional rigors of the task. In the end, as long as you are young at heart and committed to the experience, you will survive and thrive.

Can I afford it?

There are funding mechanisms in place to ensure that almost anyone who is accepted to med school can pay for it. Doing so will likely mean taking out some hefty loans, which may have a significant impact on your long-term financial planning, but it can definitely be done. In chapters 6 and 11 we will explore, in depth, the dollar value of a medical degree, why it still is a sound financial investment despite the onerous loan burden, and how to best manage your debt service while you pass through medical school and residency.

There are also a number of alternative approaches you can take that will make school virtually free. Consider a military appointment with promised service after graduation, or a National Health Service Corps grant with a commitment to placement in an underserved area once you're in practice. Such avenues are there for the taking, and with a little research, ingenuity, and careful planning, they can eliminate the onerous debt burden associated with obtaining your medical degree.

What about my life and my family?

Make no mistake—the demands of med school are very real. In order to pursue your education and your training you will, quite simply, be required to forego most nonessential aspects of your life in favor of more time and focus to study. Hobbies go largely by the wayside, and time off becomes a rare and precious commodity. Personal relationships will be continually strained by your workload.

It's not all gloom and doom, though.

Remember that hundreds of thousands of others have endured and survived this experience before you. Striving for a balanced life is a key survival tool—and one you'll constantly need to call on as a doctor. Recognizing when you need time to get away from work is crucial, and having family, friends, and loved ones who understand the demands on you and have pledged to support you along the way will be a big help. Many people end up getting married and even having children in the midst of their medical training. The only limitations are ones you impose on yourself.

In the end, no one but you can assess your true fitness and commitment to pursue medicine. The key is making your decision an informed one.

"My only words of wisdom are to know yourself fully before going into the ordeal of medicine," Pete counsels. "Those who do not know what they are seeking from the outset are unlikely to find satisfaction in today's health-care world. Realize ahead of time whether you are someone who loves knowing the most about a small subset of information or if you want to know a little about a wide range of health issues. Recognize as well the type of life you want: if you are looking for the 2.3 kids, the big house in the suburbs, the SUV, and the Wednesdays improving your golf game, those are still attainable, but you have to sacrifice much to get there. Knowing yourself is equally important for those who pursue the inner city or rural primary, grassroots-driven care of the underserved. In deciding whether or not to go into medicine, as with any other career, the key is in knowing not what you want to do, but what kind of person you want to become."

CHAPTER 2

A Road Map of the Med-School Education Process

By three methods we may learn wisdom:
first, by reflection, which is noblest;
second, by imitation, which is easiest;
and third, by experience, which is the bitterest.
—CONFUCIUS

IF YOU'RE STILL with us, you've presumably reflected on your fitness to pursue a medical degree and emerged undeterred or, even better, reassured. To most, however, med school and the experience you'll have there are shrouded in mystery. As such, the next order of business is to dispel some myths and lay bare the process with a general overview of medical education. There are many steps, many variables, and many years to the process, and this chapter will provide a blueprint for each phase of your preparation and training.

In general terms, the journey to physicianhood includes about two years of premedical prerequisites, four years of medical school, one year of internship, and at least two years of residency training before you become eligible for a specialty board certification. Understanding this road map will be key to understanding the later chapters in this book and applying its teachings to your own education. Feel free to return to these pages periodically if you find yourself lost in the maze later on.

PREPARATION AND PREREQUISITES

In order to apply to medical school you will need a bachelor's degree from an accredited college or university. You can complete any major you choose, but you also have to demonstrate your successful completion of prerequisite courses in biology, chemistry, physics, and calculus. This course work will prepare you for the Medical College Admissions Test (MCAT). The specific course requirements and a guide to the premed process are presented in the next chapter.

MED SCHOOL: FOUR YEARS, 125 FLAVORS

The first medical school in the United States was the College of Philadelphia Medical School (now known as the University of Pennsylvania School of Medicine), founded in 1765. Students enrolled for anatomical lectures and a course on the "Theory and Practice of Physik." Over time, the breadth and depth of medical knowledge grew, and by 1900 American medical schools had a relatively standard four-year curriculum followed by an internship and/or a residency. Since 1990, however, we have seen dramatic innovations in the way medical-school curricula are structured, to the point where each of the 125 currently accredited medical schools in the United States now takes its own unique approach. An overview of the different curricular formats and general philosophies of medical education follows below.

Traditional format

Today there are numerous variations in curricular structure and format in U.S. medical schools. Most, however, are still a variation on what we'll call the "traditional format." In this system, the first two years are spent almost solely dedicated to classroom course work, while the second two years are devoted to clinical work on the wards. The preclinical, didactic phase of years one and two is typically broken down into normal anatomy and physiology the first year, followed by abnormal, or diseased, physiology and therapeutics the second year. Thus, typical first-year classes might include Anatomy, Physiology, Microbiology, and Embryology, whereas typical second-year classes would include Pathology, Pathophysiology, and Pharmacology.

In the latter two years of the traditional curriculum you leave the classroom almost totally behind and receive hands-on education by rotating through the wards. Year three typically involves core rotations in internal medicine, surgery, pediatrics, obstetrics and gynecology, and sometimes various subspecialties like anesthesia. In year four, you begin to focus on the specialty in which you anticipate applying for residency. The first half of your fourth year is spent finishing prerequisites and doing acting internships in your field, often both at your home institution and at some key residency sites. You apply to residency in the fall of your fourth year, interview throughout the winter months, and spend your fourth-year spring finishing off requirements, taking elective and vacation time, and pretty much waiting with bated breath for Match Day—where you find out where you will serve your internship.

Integrated formats

Until the late 1980s, the traditional approach was the predominant format. More recently, however, medical educators and practitioners have begun to propose a more integrated didactic and clinical sequence to medical school, and as such a new era of curricular innovation has been spawned. Today, even schools with fairly traditional curricula are emphasizing some basic clinical exposure early on and throughout the four years. Additionally, instead of monolithic, didactic courses presenting a longitudinal view of a single subject across all the body's systems, there has been a push to alter the approach of the didactic curriculum as well. Some schools have turned to a systems format in which the course work is organized around a single body system. For example, a lecture block on the cardiovascular system would encompass its anatomy, physiology, pathophysiology, and pharmacology all at once.

Other schools have completely abandoned the pure didactic approach in favor of problem-based learning (PBL) in small-group environments. In this approach, a small group is presented with a clinical scenario by an instructor and, as a group, works through identifying the clinical issues, researching the pertinent data, and formulating an approach to the clinical problem. Thus, for example, a group presented with a patient who is hypertensive and recently had a heart attack might recognize they need to read about cardiac anatomy and physiology, the pathophysiology of infarction, as well as the interaction of heart, kidneys, and blood vessels in hypertension. They will need to understand not just the basis for disease and how it alters the normal structure and function of the body but also how drugs and other therapeutics are tailored to combat the diseases. In schools employing this approach, the complete spectrum of didactic knowledge is covered by the careful structuring and sequencing of these clinical scenarios.

These are just a few examples of the various versions of integrated curricular structures and formats operating in American medical schools today. While most schools offer some blend of traditional, integrated, and problem-based didactics, most schools also emphasize a particular approach to learning. As such, in developing your list of med schools during your application process, consider which format best suits your learning style. Do you need the structure and rigor of large classroom lectures, or are you better in small, creative, self-directed groups? With sufficient research, you can find the perfect curriculum to suit your preferred learning style.

M.D. Versus D.O. Programs

It is worth pausing here to clarify the distinction between the two different types of medical schools in the United States and the different degrees they offer. The majority of U.S. medical schools feature the traditional allopathic curriculum, covering the spectrum of human pathology and its treatment via surgery, medicines, and therapeutics. These schools award the M.D. (Medical Doctor) degree. Osteopathic medical schools offer an alternate and complementary approach providing the same training and experience in medicine, surgery, and therapeutics while also featuring specialized training in manipulative techniques. These therapeutic techniques are more closely aligned to chiropractic manipulations and seek to treat both musculoskeletal and physiologic disease by adjusting the skeletal structure of the body, thereby returning it to normal, functional alignment, relieving symptoms and restoring health. These medical schools award the D.O. (Doctor of Osteopathy) degree. All medical specialties accept both M.D. and D.O. physicians, and D.O. physicians are fully trained and accredited in all aspects of traditional allopathic medicine.

Since the vast majority (approximately 94 percent) of physicians are graduates of allopathic schools, this has traditionally been the more competitive route through medical school. Yet osteopathic students also attend school for four years and then typically either matriculate into a standard residency or do an additional year of osteopathic clinical training before beginning residency. There are some osteopathic-specific residencies, but most residencies accept both M.D. and D.O. candidates, though not always with equal enthusiasm.

"I learned about osteopathic medicine by working in a clinic that was staffed by both M.D.s and D.O.s," Kate explains. "I found that D.O.s had a little something extra to offer to their patients—namely, a whole body philosophy and manual manipulation. I learned more about this technique and the theories behind it while working at the clinic. This provided me with the exposure that I needed to make the decision to pursue an emergency-medicine career as a D.O.

"As a D.O. in the emergency department, I often find that I do not have time to perform manual manipulation. This is disappointing, but I do educate my patients on what they can do for themselves to help their recovery from their musculoskeletal complaints. Empowering patients is just as important as treating them.

"Prior to entering my allopathic EM residency, I chose to complete a Traditional Osteopathic Rotating Internship. This was essentially a prelim year (medicine, pediatrics, ob, surgery, emergency medicine, etc.) with osteopathic manual manipulation entwined throughout the year, allowing me to develop my manual manipulation skills. I think this is very important if you are a D.O. who ends up in an allopathic residency program. Not only did it help me develop my osteopathic skills, but it allowed me to mature as a clinician. As an emergency physician, you are expected to know a little bit about everything. This extra year has helped me to do just that—which benefits not only my education but more importantly my patients."

Although unfounded, there is a fairly pervasive perception in the allopathic community that osteopathic training is somehow inferior. Allopathic medical schools do tend to be more difficult to get into, and hence osteopathic schools are considered by many to be a second-tier alternative. Fair or not, it is important to be aware of this perception in advance, because when it comes time to pursue residency and career options, osteopaths can find themselves at a competitive disadvantage in the marketplace.

M.D./Ph.D. Programs

For the truly stout of heart, many schools offer an M.D./Ph.D. track. The M.D./Ph.D. is primarily a research-focused program in which the graduating candidate will earn both a Doctor of Medicine and a Doctor of Science degree. Typically, the curriculum is modified such that you take some additional classes in research methodology during your first two preclinical years and then take at least a year between the preclinical and clinical phases to focus solely on a major, doctoral-level research project and dissertation. An M.D./Ph.D. is an exceptional degree and offers entry into the hallowed community of high-level academic and clinical research. There are, of course, many active researchers who do not have Ph.D.s, but possessing the joint degree clearly defines you as a specialist in your field.

"The Match" and Applying to Residency

The process of applying to residency is drastically different from applying to medical school. All institutions in the United States that offer medical residencies belong to the National Resident Matching Program (NRMP). This body links residency applicants to residency programs. The system tries to match the strength of your desire for a program with the program's desire to have you as a resident.

Here's a thumbnail sketch of how it works:

In the fall of your fourth year of medical school, you will apply to residency programs in your chosen field. Residency programs vary in structure and format, but are universally composed of at least one initial year of internship followed by some number of years of residency thereafter. Some institutions integrate the internship, or first year, into their residency program, such that you will start on day one as a member of that program and graduate the requisite number of years later from the same place. Other residency programs start in postgraduate year two (PGY-2), meaning that you'll be required to apply to, match to, and complete an internship elsewhere before matriculating into the residency program you've selected.

Once you've chosen your field of specialty, done your research, selected your programs, and applied, you wait for an invitation to be interviewed. In February of your fourth year of med school, once the interviewing process is complete, you submit your match list to the

NRMP. On this list you will sequentially rank the programs that interviewed you from your first choice to your last choice. Around the same time, all the residency programs in the country assemble a similar match list, listing in sequential order the candidates they would most like to have as residents. A giant computer at the NRMP uses a complex algorithm to sort through these lists and match candidates to positions.

On or around March 18 of your fourth year of medical school you will receive notification from the NRMP of your match. This match represents a binding contract, so where you match, you go. In many fields and many programs there are more candidates than positions, meaning that you may or may not achieve your number one choice. Careful construction of your match list will help ensure that you match somewhere you want to go.

If all of this has just devolved into a big blur for you, don't worry. Remember that this chapter is just an overview of the entire experience. We'll tell you everything you need to know about applying to residency programs and surviving the match in part five of this book.

INTERNSHIP, RESIDENCY, AND BEYOND

Most doctors cite their internship as the most memorable year of their medical training. Not only will your year as an intern likely be one of the busiest of your life, it will also represent your rite of passage from book-toting, bewildered medical student to competent clinician. It is for most people an exciting, terrifying, exhausting time. That said, in the current climate of work-hours reform and concern for physician wellness, internships across the country are increasingly focused on providing a less hellacious and more manageable experience.

So what is this thing called "internship," anyway?

As an intern you will, for the first time, assume primary responsibility for patient care. As with each stage in the training process, the biggest transition in an internship will be a new and significantly higher level of patient-care responsibility. As a third-year medical student, you will have struggled to figure out how to complete a thorough history and physical exam (H & P) and write a decent chart note. As a fourth-year medical student during your acting intern rotation, you will have been asked to take on a larger portion of the care of a few patients at a time. During your internship, however, you will be expected to carry a significant daily patient load, to cross-cover entire services of patients you may not be familiar with while on call at night, and to report directly to senior residents and attending physicians on your clinical assessments and therapeutic plans. It's a big step up in responsibility and workload. But the reality is that you have a team of senior residents and attendings who are prepared to support and shepherd you through the process. Furthermore, you'll also have talented nursing staff at the bedside—people who will teach you a great deal and save you from yourself during those late-night crises when a patient goes into a death spiral and it seems like you're the only one around!

At the end of your intern year, you will make another leap in responsibility. If your internship was separate from your residency, you may be moving to a new place and starting out with all new colleagues. But even if you're in an integrated program, your second year will be one in which you take on a larger patient load and have more involvement in leading clinical teams and overseeing interns and medical students. Chances are, shortly after you start your residency, you will look into the wide eyes of one of your interns or med students and realize just how far you've come.

The number of years of residency training varies from specialty to specialty. At a minimum you will complete one year of internship and two years of residency. No matter how long your training program is, you will continue to progress in your clinical responsibilities and oversight levels from year to year. By the time you become a senior resident you may be elected to or designated a chief resident. As a chief, you will continue to fulfill your ordinary clinical duties but will also undertake a full slate of administrative duties and oversight responsibilities.

Once again, remember that this chapter is merely intended to provide an overview. We handle the specific details of residency and provide all the strategies for optimizing your residency experience in part six of this book.

MEDICAL LICENSING

You must obtain a U.S. Medical License in order to practice medicine in the United States. To do this you must pass all three steps of the United States Medical Licensing Exam (USMLE). Typically you will take Step 1 of the test after the first two preclinical years in medical school, Step 2 during your fourth year of medical school, and Step 3 after one year of postgraduate training (i.e., internship). After you've passed all three Step Exams, you will have completed national certification and can apply for a state license to practice medicine. Thankfully, this is just a matter of filing paperwork. You are not required to pass any additional tests to get licensed in different states.

During your residency training, you will probably work under a provisional license of the hospital and residency program, so you don't need to complete your medical licensing application process until you actually complete your training. Getting all of your licensing credentials while still in training, however, will allow you to moonlight—that is, get paid for picking up extra shifts at facilities outside your training program. Some residencies restrict moonlighting, while others encourage it as a way to expand your clinical experience. Whatever the case, moonlighting can be an important source of additional income to the financially strapped resident.

Successfully completing each USMLE Step Exam is a major rite of passage on the long road through medical school. The USMLE Step Exams are intense, comprehensive experiences that require extensive study. Step 1 covers the full spectrum of medical knowledge and will truly test your ability to regurgitate and apply the preclinical material from the first two years of med school. Step 2 is based on clinical scenarios and will test your clinical decision making; it includes the Objective Structured Clinical Exam (OSCE)—a live demonstration of your clinical skills on actors trained as simulated patients. On this portion of the Step 2 Exam, you will be asked to demonstrate your interview skills, your physical-examination skills, and your clinical decision-making skills in a simulated clinical encounter. Finally, Step 3 attempts to test your more advanced clinical decision-making and medical-management skills. It also includes a computerized, case-based simulation component.

We'll review each of the Step Exams as they come up chronologically in the chapters ahead.

Fellowship Training

While in residency, you may decide you wish to continue your training to subspecialize within your discipline. To do this, you will have to complete a fellowship—typically an additional one to four years of focused, high-level training. Most fields offer some form of subspecialty training. For example, cardiology is a subspecialty fellowship of internal medicine. Similarly, cardiothoracic is a subspecialty of general surgery, and neonatology is a subspecialty of pediatrics. At the end of most fellowships you will be eligible for subspecialty board certification.

Board Certification

The long road to physicianhood ends with the completion of your board certification. After graduating from your residency or fellowship you will be eligible to sit for your specialty or subspecialty boards. This is typically a two-day written examination created by a board of specialists in your field. Many specialties also require an oral board exam. In the oral exam, you will spend one or two days facing clinical case scenarios presented by a trained examiner, and you will be expected to verbally walk through the case, manage the patient, and reach a diagnosis. This is essentially a more basic version of the OSCE designed to test your reasoning skills on your feet.

CHAPTER 3

Surviving Premed

If you want the rainbow, you gotta put up with the rain.
—DOLLY PARTON

IT IS UNDENIABLE that a solid foundation in the fundamentals of science is imperative to your subsequent medical education. That said, the set of hurdles imposed by college premed programs is more a means to weed out those not fanatically dedicated to medicine than it is the wellspring of foundational knowledge required of physicians and clinical scientists. Thus, the goal in premed is simply to overcome this important first hurdle in your medical education and arrive on the other side with your enthusiasm intact. The best way to accomplish this is to arm yourself with an understanding of the process, keep your eye on your goals, and be creative wherever you can.

Let's look at what classes are required and what you can do to excel in them, either as an undergraduate or as a postbaccalaureate student.

THE PREMED REQUIREMENTS

The Association of American Medical Colleges (AAMC) publishes a guide, *Medical School Admission Requirements (MSAR),* that is a worthwhile investment at the outset of your premed studies. This guide, available from the AAMC Web site (www.aamc.org/medical schools.htm), details the basic course requirements, which include:

Physics	2 semesters
Biology	2 semesters
Chemistry—Inorganic	2 semesters
Chemistry—Organic	2 semesters
Calculus	1 semester

If you took Advanced Placement (AP) classes or International Baccalaureate (IB) classes in high school, you may be eligible to receive college-level credit and thus place out of some of these courses. If you have a solid, foundational understanding of biology, physics, inorganic chemistry, and calculus, we highly recommend placing out of as many of these requirements as possible, since the general premed curriculum will otherwise consume approximately one-fourth of your college course load and require a very significant obligation of time, effort, and dedication.

PREMED AS AN UNDERGRADUATE

If you're still an undergraduate and didn't place out of any of these courses, you may find yourself staring at the above list of classes and wondering how you can possibly cram that list into four years already jam-packed with your other curricular requirements.

Relax. With a little bit of creative planning, you can prevent your premed requirements from eclipsing your liberal arts education and precluding the normal pleasures of college life.

Your primary task will be to avoid the myopic sense of drudgery that the premed curriculum instills and remember that college offers an astounding opportunity to delve deeply into a vast array of subjects. Focusing solely on the premed curriculum or choosing a major based on it at the expense of other interests may stultify and embitter you and deny you those nonscientific exposures and ideas that could well be *the* creative spark in your med-school application.

To strike the critical balance between courses you *must* take and the courses you *want* to take, you have several tools at your disposal. First, your college or university almost certainly employs a premed advisor. Get to know this person early in your life on campus. Not only will this person be able to offer important insight and guidance about the premed process, he or she will also be a critical source for a letter of recommendation someday. Ask about the typical sequence of classes, who the best professors are, when to take what, and which courses should not be taken concurrently. Find out what the most challenging classes are and how best to manage them. Write out a four-year master semester schedule and pencil in all the required classes. Now as you go about matching up your other nonpremed classes semester by semester, you'll be able to sense what your premed workload will be and how best to fit the pieces of the puzzle together.

"I took all of my premed classes as a freshman and sophomore in college," Adam recalls. "In a way I wish I had spread them out, as I probably would have been a bit more focused and done better in them."

Surviving and thriving in the premed curriculum

Keep several key points in mind as you approach each of your premed classes. First, your performance in these classes will be closely scrutinized when you apply to medical school, so you should devote the necessary time, energy, and focus to them to ensure that you do your best. This does not mean that if you don't maintain a 4.0 average in these classes you should order up a copy of *Law School Confidential* and reconsider your options. What it does mean is that these are classes that must be taken seriously.

And what does *that* mean?

Get organized early and stay organized. Stay on top of your problem sets, labs, and upcoming tests, and get extra help at the first sign of trouble. Most schools have built-in premed tutoring programs that can provide some additional one-on-one teaching time that can really make a difference, often at no additional cost to you. Second, remember that while these classes are billed as integral to your medical education, they are really just the primary training for your first big med-school hurdle—the MCAT. We strongly recommend buying an MCAT review book as you begin your journey through the premed curriculum and reading through the relevant material as you proceed through a given course. As you prepare for your exams in college, use a bank of MCAT-prep questions to hone your skills on a particular topic. This will help emphasize and reinforce the range and depth of topics typically covered on the MCAT and get you in the habit of using review books in conjunction with studying for classes— a tactic you will want to use again and again in medical school.

You must also strive to find personal relevance, interest, or real-world applicability in the premed curriculum. You're learning stuff at a fundamental, often abstract level, but all of this stuff applies one way or another. Seek out examples of those applications. When reading about Pascal's gas law, try to seek out some examples from pulmonary physiology; when grappling with the Henderson Hasselbach equation and acid-base chemistry, think about how these topics apply to buffering systems in the blood. Specific references to clinical medicine in your classroom lectures will, unfortunately, likely be few and far between, so focus and invigorate your studies by drumming up your own clinically oriented examples for projects and papers. Most professors will be happy to help you explore the clinical application of your basic science studies during office hours. Make the time to find these connections.

Finally, a last piece of advice: you'll be studying medicine in one form or another for the rest of your life. The long road ahead features years of medical school, residency, and a lifetime of learning as a clinician to pursue the nuances of science in medicine. Take advantage of your four years as an undergraduate to become *educated*. Don't succumb to the urge to follow the well-beaten path of the premed drones, blindly pursuing a biology major, volunteering at the university hospital, becoming an EMT, and surviving all of your other curriculum requirements with Cliffs Notes and canned outlines. Taking this approach will render you colorless and indistinguishable from thousands of other med-school applicants a few years down the road, and it will cheat you of one of the most formative experiences of your lifetime.

Take time to explore the curriculum and to find new horizons in areas you didn't even know existed. Test your commitment to the medical profession. Yes, it will be a juggling act to seriously pursue other areas of interest while hammering away at the premed classes. In the end, though, it will pay off not only in making you a well-educated person but also in extending the scope of your med-school application into important nonmedical arenas that, as Dr. Friedman notes in the foreword to this book, are especially attractive to today's admissions committees searching for well-rounded, "human" applicants.

Make sure your explorations extend beyond your courses as well. College is filled with unparalleled opportunities to get involved in all manner of activities, projects, travels, and groups. Find out if you can get involved in the local ski patrol. Scan the bulletin boards of various departments looking for assistants for far-flung trips to do research or offer humanitarian assistance. Remember that everyone's med-school application will have the exact same premed classes, probably with similar grades. Look for ways to extend yourself with a different major or a different course load, and challenge yourself with a different array of experiences, and thus distinguish yourself as someone with the independent mind and the adventuresome, inquisitive spirit most sought after by med-school admissions committees.

> I decided during the beginning of my senior year that I was going to take one year off after college before attending medical school. I found a nonprofit group based in Utah that ran Peace Corps–like programs in countries around the world. I ended up working for them in Bolivia, spending seven months living with the Aymara Indians.
>
> —Adam

PREMED AS A POSTBAC

For those of you going back to satisfy your premed requirements after college, the road is a bit trickier. Chances are, you have a job and a life, and as such you may be less able to simply drop everything and dedicate yourself solely to banging out these difficult classes in rapid succession. As someone already out in the working world, you may have less tolerance for busywork, and the idea of returning to entry-level undergraduate classes will likely be considerably less appealing than it was your freshman year, especially without the keg parties.

"When you've been out a while, it seems bizarre to be back in an academic environment, and it was difficult for me to adjust," Ben notes. "That being said, I think most of us who went back to complete premed requirements tended to have a broader perspective on what was important and what was not."

"I served on my medical school's admissions committee for two years," Adam says, "and I can say with assurance that there is no disadvantage to taking time between college and medical school. An applicant can show sufficient interest in medicine regardless of his or her path to medical school."

There are actually some important potential advantages to doing a postbac premed plan. First, you will be older and wiser than your classmates who come straight from college. You've likely worked or traveled a bit and subsequently decided to go back and pursue medicine after an assortment of real-life experiences. This means you now have a focused goal, and more advanced and varied skills to achieve it. You're better able to prioritize and keep the forest in view while working among the trees. Since you've already completed college, your sole focus can be your premed studies and making sure you shine.

Second, and perhaps most important, you have maturity, experience, and perspective on your side. You've arrived at medicine's doorstep on a path whose tried-and-tested alternatives led you to the conclusion that your passion and future lie in medicine. This informed decision making should provide an important source of staying power, passion, and focus as you grind through the premed classes.

"I think it is an enormous advantage to experience the world before plunging into the myopic existence of medicine," Pete explains. "The perspectives you gain from working in the real world with real people are invaluable in providing understanding and compassionate care to whatever community you end up practicing medicine in. That appreciation of the people you work with is so important, as is the self-knowledge that comes from pursuing alternative paths before settling into medicine. The flip sides to this, however, are multiple. First, it's much more physically and emotionally draining to go through the rigors of residency as an older individual, particularly if you have children or a partner as part of your life at that point. Second, you realize how cushy a forty-hour workweek really is and can personally contrast that with the eighty-plus hours per week you work in the hospital as a resident and sometimes as an attending."

I believe quite strongly that it is an advantage to take time off between undergrad and med school. Some will say it makes you a stronger applicant, mostly because you have something else to talk about during your interviews. More important, though, I think it makes med school and residency easier. When you are sitting in the library at midnight during the middle of your first year in medical school or on call for the tenth time in three weeks during your internship, you won't be haunted by the what-ifs that bother the kids who went straight through. You will have been out there in the real world. You will know firsthand how boring a staff meeting can be or how absolutely humiliating it can be to work in a cubical for a boss who is, at best, a moron. You know that you never want to have a regular nine-to-five job when being a doctor would be so much more fun.

—Chris

Where to complete your premed requirements

Where you take your premed classes is relatively unimportant. Some people return to their undergraduate institution, which has the advantage of producing a uniform academic record. Some people enroll in one of the many intensive postbac premed programs around the country. These programs, which are familiar to and typically well-regarded by med schools, are designed to be factories to crank you out through the premed process. Others simply take the classes at whatever institution is closest to their jobs and families, allowing them to continue working and living in the same area while completing the requirements. The Association of American Medical Colleges (AAMC) Web site (www.aamc.org) has a listing of every public and private premed program in the country to help you choose the program that works best for your situation.

How to structure your course work as a postbac

Once you enroll in a postbac program, you should immediately schedule a meeting with the premed advisor. This is an absolutely critical step. Planning the sequence of your courses as a postbac can be a confusing process, since restrictions on when and how you take each class vary at different institutions. Time and financial constraints may also limit your window of opportunity to pursue and complete your prerequisites. Do not end up being forced to delay your MCAT administration or completing your applications because you were unable to fulfill a requirement in time!

During your meeting with your premed advisor, declare your intentions, review your undergraduate record, and get advice on how to chart the course. You should also contact the premed advisor from your former undergraduate institution (if it is different from where you're taking your premed classes) to coordinate your efforts. If you do this, the premed advisor from your undergraduate institution can speak about the merits of the balance of your undergraduate record in a letter of recommendation from the premed committee of that school—which will enhance your record.

As a postbac, you should also coordinate your studies with your MCAT preparation. You're back in school for one reason and one reason only—to bang out your prereqs and pass the MCAT. Get a good MCAT review book on day one and start targeting your postbac studies toward the concepts covered in the book. When you're reviewing for your exams in school, use a bank of MCAT practice questions to hone your skills. Read the next section on taking the MCAT carefully, and schedule your study and test taking to fit into your compressed premed curriculum.

Finally, it may have been a while since you've been enrolled in full-time classes. Be honest with yourself and evaluate your progress as you go. If you feel like you're slipping or getting into academic trouble, put ego aside and ask for help. Avail yourself of tutoring, get extra help from your teaching assistants, or check in with your professor during office hours to remedy the situation promptly.

CHAPTER 4

Beating the MCAT

At college age, you can tell who is the best at taking tests . . .
but you can't tell who the best people are.
That worries the hell out of me.
—BARNABY C. KEENEY

AS YOU'VE PROBABLY heard, the MCAT is one of those monolithic, life-altering, gatekeeper experiences. But is it really as horrible as people say it is? Let's separate fact from fiction.

The MCAT will be, without a doubt, the longest and most difficult exam you will have taken to date. Your pent-up anxiety after months of studying, and the overwhelming sense of anxiety of everyone around you, will add significantly to the challenge. In the weeks and days leading up to the administration of the exam, it will seem like it's all anyone can talk about, and that the only thing worse than actually studying for the MCAT is the paralyzing fear that this one seven-hour exam could actually stymie your dream of becoming a doctor.

Don't let it.

There are kernels of reality to the MCAT hype, but if you take to heart the advice that follows, the experience need not be one that lands you in therapy. This chapter will familiarize you with the basics of the test and arm you with a strategy and some useful resources. There are literally hundreds of MCAT preparatory books available on the market, and this book is not intended to be another one of those. Our goal with respect to your MCAT preparation is simply to dispel some myths and provide a direction for your intensive, independent preparation for the exam.

"It is just something you have to do," Kate counsels. "Get through it."

What the Test Is All About

As in nearly all academic admissions processes, medical schools seek a universal objective measure of their candidates. Just as the SAT was your ticket into college, the MCAT is your pass into medical school. And, just like the SAT or any other standardized test, the MCAT is highly imperfect.

Its makers, the Association of American Medical Colleges (AAMC), claim that the MCAT is "designed to assess problem solving, critical thinking, and writing skills in addition to the examinee's knowledge of science concepts and principles prerequisite to the study of medicine." Proponents of the MCAT, mostly within the admissions world, claim that MCAT scores correlate well with students' actual success in medical school. And as you might expect, there are many who question this assertion and examples too numerous to recount of people who underperformed on the MCAT and went on to become stars in the medical profession. That said, like it or not, performing at least passably well on the MCAT *will* be a make-it-or-break-it factor in your application. Schools may claim they don't screen on MCAT scores, but the reality is that with too many qualified applicants for too few slots, most med schools do, in fact, prescreen applicants on some objective criteria, often including the MCAT score.

So how should you approach this beast?

While you do need a solid base of science knowledge in order to score well on the test, the truth is that like any standardized test the MCAT does a better job of assessing how well you take standardized tests. Preparing for the test thus becomes a game of rehearsing the basic information you need as background to the test, and then mastering the games the test makers play with the questions. The test is comprehensive, but it actually covers a fairly limited set of specific information from a wide range of subjects. With enough time and a direction, you can review and master this information. The trick is training yourself to become an expert at *taking* the MCAT. This will mean understanding the types of questions asked, knowing and learning to recognize the tricks, and, you guessed it—practice, practice, and more practice.

By the end of this preparatory ordeal you will feel like you are eating, living, and breathing test questions. You'll do so many practice exams you'll feel like a day without multiple-choice questions is somehow lacking. And when you reach that point, you'll be ready. But you're a long way from there now, so read on.

Let's start by looking at how the test is put together and how it is administered.

How the Test Is Structured

The MCAT has approximately 214 multiple-choice questions and two writing sections. It is broken down into four separate sections. When all is said and done, you will spend seven hours taking the actual test, with two short breaks and a lunch hour interspersed in that time. Count on a full eight-hour day when you consider getting there, getting registered, and getting oriented.

Each section of the MCAT covers a different subject area or skill set. The sections, and the typical structure of those sections, are listed in the following chart.

MCAT Section	Questions	Duration
Physical Sciences	77 questions	100 minutes
—Break—		10 minutes
Verbal Reasoning	60 questions	85 minutes
—Lunch—		60 minutes
Biological Sciences	77 questions	100 minutes
—Break—		10 minutes
Writing Sample	2 essays	60 minutes

The question formats are fairly typical of any long standardized test. The physical and biological sciences sections are all multiple-choice questions, often referring to a reading passage relevant to the subject matter. The verbal reasoning section is also all multiple-choice, but these questions relate exclusively to fairly extensive reading passages from the social and natural sciences, as well as the humanities. In the verbal reasoning section you are not tested on your science and humanities knowledge but on your reading comprehension, reasoning, and critical-thinking skills. Finally, the essay section is composed of two brief topic statements. For each statement, you are instructed to write a roughly one-page responsive essay to "elicit a unified, coherent, first-draft essay exploring the meaning and implications of the statement."

The AAMC draws on many resources to help write MCAT questions. Contributors include the AAMC staff, medical-school admissions officers, medical-school faculties, college faculties, and practicing physicians. As with all standardized tests, your test will contain some new, experimental questions. Your answers to these questions will not be reported as part of your score but rather used to evaluate their merit for inclusion on future MCATs.

HOW THE TEST IS SCORED, AND WHAT THE RESULTS MEAN

You will receive an individual score from 1 (lowest) to 15 (highest) on each of the three multiple-choice sections. You receive full credit for the questions you got right and no deduction for the questions you got wrong, so guessing is always preferable to leaving questions unanswered. Your raw score for a given section is then converted to the 15-point scale. The actual conversion formula is a complicated and closely guarded secret that takes into account variations in the types of questions used on the actual test you take, and evens out minor variations in test administration, personal performance, and test quality. Your scaled score will then be used to derive percentile ranks specific to your test date and to the year you took the test. These are perhaps the most useful numbers to the admissions committees, since they are the best evaluation of your test aptitude relative to that of your peers taking the same test at the same time. Medical schools will total the numeric scores on the three multiple-choice sections and use this as an estimate of your overall performance on the exam.

The writing sample is scored a bit differently. Each essay is read by a reviewer who assigns a series of numeric scores that reflect your organization and style in the essay. The numeric scores from both essays are then converted to a single-letter score from J (lowest) to T (highest). Why the AAMC chose the letters J through T is one of life's great mysteries. Nonetheless, your score report will bear one of these letters as the score for your writing samples.

So what do these scores mean, and how can you judge how well you did?

Almost all schools now require the MCAT for admissions. Most will publish a range or average score for their entering classes, giving you a general sense of how strongly they weigh MCAT performance and, indirectly, how competitive their candidates are. In 2004 the mean cumulative score for the combined April/August administrations was 24.6 with the individual means being 8.1 for physical sciences, 8.0 for verbal reasoning, and 8.5 for biological sciences. The average writing sample score was an O, with prominent peaks at the M and Q levels. In general you should hope to score at least 9 to 12 on each section.

A general rule of thumb over the years has been that a combined numeric score of 30 gets your application over the threshold and into the files under active consideration at most schools. This means you could, theoretically, bomb the verbal with a 4 and ace the physical and biological sciences with 13s respectively and still make the 30 cutoff. Med-school admissions committees **do** review the individual section scores, though, so if you really bomb one section, it will get noticed.

The writing section is generally not used as a screening tool. If you absolutely bomb the writing section, schools may look to other indicators in your academic record and your application essay for further information about your writing ability. If you do poorly here, it won't kill you. On the other hand, an exceptional writing sample score and a strong application essay will be definite pluses in your application. Anything in between will probably neither hurt nor help you.

PREPARING FOR THE MCAT

There is an infinite array of strategies for preparing for the MCAT that all boil down to three essential ingredients: time, determination, and hard work. The exact quantities of each that will be required of you will depend on your past test-taking performance, your anxiety level, your time constraints, and the freshness of your premed coursework. Of the essential ingredients, time will be the most critical to get a handle on early.

First a basic, seemingly obvious, but absolutely crucial point: never *ever* take the MCAT cold!

The test is simply too long, too complicated, too comprehensive, and fundamentally too important to take lightly. Even if you have a long history of acing standardized tests, it will be well worth your while to spend some time understanding the scope of the information covered on the MCAT and the structure of the test. Preparing can only improve your scores, which will improve your candidacy in the highly competitive med-school admissions process, and, thus, likely reduce your anxiety in the long run.

You should start preparing for the MCAT and developing a study strategy at least a year ahead of the time that you anticipate applying to medical school. This will give you sufficient time to self-evaluate, develop a study plan, and remedy any weakness you may have. Most students allot approximately three months of *dedicated* study time to preparing for the MCAT. Since the test is offered only twice, in April and August of each year, you'll have to pick the test date that works best for you and coordinate your study schedule accordingly. Most people take the test in April of their junior year, since they will then receive their scores during the summer and can evaluate their results before the August/September application crunch time.

"I took the MCAT as an undergrad," Deb recalls. "Then, when I decided to reapply for medical school, I unfortunately had to take it again. I think there was a five-year limit for how long your scores were valid, and of course I was past that. That was my biggest woe of reapplying. I remember sitting on my porch in the middle of summer trying to review calculus and physics, which I didn't really understand when I took them in college and surely didn't remember six years later after not having to use them or think about them in any way, shape, or form in my job or everyday life. That was a drag!"

Getting started and doing a diagnostic test

When you begin formulating your study plan, start by gathering the basic information about the test. The AAMC Web site (www.aamc.org) provides excruciatingly detailed information on the test as well as some downloadable banks of sample questions. You should also consult your premed advisor or premed office for their list of recommended resources for study. Finally, there's a wide array of MCAT preparation books that offer review information, test-taking strategies, and sample tests. We provide our recommended list of study aids in the appendix.

Once you get a basic feel for the exam's scope and coverage, you should think about taking a diagnostic practice test. This needn't be a simulation of the entire MCAT, only a representative exam covering each of the sections. You can use the AAMC versions or any of the commercially available versions of practice tests.

Before you start this first practice test, take this fact to heart: you will probably *bomb* it.

It's okay. Don't panic.

This test is designed just to give you a feel for the questions, a sense of how they test the knowledge, and, most important, a list of areas you need to improve on. Your scores will get better, so hang in there. You're only just beginning.

The results of your diagnostic practice test will, no doubt, help you assess the time commitment required for your preparation. If you're historically a strong standardized-test taker and you fared well on the diagnostic test, you can probably focus your preparation on taking more practice exams and reviewing the subtle concepts that may help you ratchet up your score another notch. If you're disappointed in your performance on the diagnostic test, it's time for the next crucial assessment: is it the test, the substantive concepts, or both that are tripping you up?

Look through the answers for your diagnostic test and scrutinize the written explanations. Try to honestly assess whether you got a question wrong because you didn't know the information, or because the question was asked in such a way that you failed to apply or recognize facts you already knew. If it's the former, you'll need to prioritize your preparation plan first on a review of substantive material, and then doing more practice tests. If it's the latter, you should still review substance, but you should focus more of your preparation on perfecting test-taking strategies.

Study strategies: deciding between self-study and commercial review courses

Armed with a sense of your initial performance and a direction for your study plan, you must next decide how to best achieve your goals and how to schedule yourself to meet these objectives. You will ultimately have to design your own preparation plan that suits your specific study needs. It is critical that your plan include a coherent structure and regular schedule. Preparing for the MCAT is a substantial undertaking. You must develop a review road map and tie it to a calendar of regular, blocked-out study times that you can adhere to. You also need to build in frequent practice exams to help gauge your progress and refine your studies.

One of the first essential decisions you face in formulating your plan is whether to prepare independently or to use a commercial review class. There are numerous commercial MCAT-preparation classes available (Kaplan, Princeton Review, and so forth) that offer thorough, intensive review and study plans for the exam. These programs hold regular classes that extensively and intensively review the required subject matter and also offer specialized, computer-driven training on subject blocks and question types, as well as full-length practice exams so you can monitor your performance as you go. Most companies offer private tutoring and online review options as well. The average cost of one of these review courses is around $1,500 to $2,000.

> I took a Princeton Review course and took about three full-length sample tests. It was pretty helpful in understanding what the test was going to be all about. It is a very specific kind of exam, and knowing the kinds of questions you'll face and the time pressure you'll be under is crucial.
>
> —Adam

The comprehensive, structured review provided by these classes is useful, and it will likely help highlight substantive gaps and otherwise clear the cobwebs on some important concepts you may not have covered for several years. The proctored, full-length, professionally scored practice tests also provide the most realistic simulation of the actual exam.

The downside to these review programs is that you may find yourself spending hours in classes reviewing material you already know. These courses can also breed anxiety, causing you and your review-course classmates to feed off each other's stress and escalate difficulties out of proportion. Finally, the one-size-fits-all approach means that if you are stuck on certain concepts, you may have to skim them and supplement with private tutoring or extra sessions in order to keep up with the class.

> I also took the Princeton Review and found it very helpful. I don't think it was the particular class, but more the way it helped focus and encourage studying. It was worth the investment.
>
> —Ben

In the end you will have to make your own decision about what best suits your needs and your learning style. For applicants more distant from the substantive knowledge of premed class work, a rapid review course may be just what the doctor ordered. Similarly, if you fear that you will lack the substantial discipline required to establish and adhere to a regular study schedule, having classes to go to and scheduled practice tests to measure your progress may be just the structure and incentive you need. For those with the ability to maintain a disciplined study schedule, however, a self-study plan may be just as good.

Practice, practice, practice!

Whatever your approach, we cannot emphasize enough the critical role that regular practice tests must play in your study plan. Remember, the MCAT is a game, not a true evaluation of your substantive knowledge. The *only* way to get better at taking the test and learning its tricks is to practice.

But simply taking practice tests is not enough.

Once you've completed a practice test, it is critical that you go through each question and understand either why you got the question right or why you got it wrong. If a conceptual issue gave you trouble, add the topic to a running list of substantive *concepts* requiring your further review. If you misinterpreted the question or failed to uncover the trick in its logic, flag it on your running list of question *types* that give you trouble. The MCAT uses a very finite array of question types. If you can identify which types of questions give you trouble, you can focus your studies on tips and tricks for handling those types of questions. The trick is to learn from the practice tests you take. Don't just take a bunch of tests, as the repetition only gets you so far. Examine your mistakes carefully, and you'll learn from them and get stronger. Don't just study hard—study smart!

The single hardest part of your MCAT preparation will be sustaining the commitment required to prepare properly. There will be countless times when you don't feel like studying but know you should. There will be concepts that you tell yourself you understand, but you know you really don't. These are the times to redouble your efforts and make sure you stay dedicated to the mission. As you take and critically evaluate more and more practice tests, you should see a gradual but steady improvement in your practice test scores.

During my senior year I studied using a handful of review books. I took the test seriously, but I thought it would be like all the other high-stress exams I had experienced in college. I spent almost no time preparing for the verbal section. I took a few practice tests out of a cheap test book and convinced myself I was well prepared. In reality, I discovered in an alarming fashion how incredibly unprepared I was. On test day I found myself rushing to finish sections and actually ran out of time before I was able to finish the verbal section, scoring a 6. I did only a mediocre job with the rest of the test, scoring a 10 on the physical sciences and an 8 on the biology section. With a total score of 24, I knew getting into any med school would be almost impossible. I had a conflict that coming summer that prevented me from retaking the MCAT in August. I still believed I had what it took to become a physician, so I made a decision at that point, ten full months ahead of time, not to underestimate the test again.

On October 1 that same year I started studying full-time for the MCAT, which was still six months away. Often I would spend several hours a night and most of the weekend going over review material. In January I enrolled in the Kaplan course, and by the end of March I had used every piece of material they had for review at least once. I went everywhere with my index cards. Interestingly, at no point did I feel I was learning any new material. Often I would find myself helping my Kaplan instructor explain concepts to our class. I already understood the science that was behind the questions. What I *was* learning was how to take the MCAT. My strategy worked well, and I did substantially better the second time around, scoring a 9 in the verbal, 12 on the biology, and a 13 on the physical sciences section, for a total of 34, a ten-point increase over my initial score. Trust me, I was no smarter a year later. If anything, I had lost some of the knowledge from my undergrad studies, as I was another year removed from it. I was, however, a well-trained test taker, and I found myself avoiding many of the pitfalls of the test that had so significantly slowed me down the year before.

—Chris

REGISTERING FOR AND TAKING THE TEST

Registration for the MCAT is done through the AAMC Web site (www.aamc.org/students/mcat/). The test is offered in April and August of each year at specific test sites throughout the United States. The AAMC recommends you take the test eighteen months before your anticipated matriculation. That's probably ideal but certainly isn't mandatory. Many people take the April test in the spring before their October application deadline. You can register for the MCAT twelve weeks prior to the test.

Registration costs $210, with fee assistance available for those in need. Starting in 2005, you had the option of registering for a computer-based exam instead of a paper-based exam. Most students are more familiar with paper-based exams, so this is their natural preference. However, you should be aware that the USMLE Step Exams, the standardized licensing exams you'll take in med school, are all computer-based. If you're comfortable working on a computer screen, you may wish to consider this format. If you choose this option, however, be sure to practice on the computer rather than just on paper, as the computer-based format has a very different feel and presents some strategic limitations.

When you register, you will be given a list of potential test sites closest to your area, and you will be asked to rank these sites in preferential order. You will be assigned a test site according to your list and the test center's availability. In urban areas, there are a lot of potential candidates who will all be taking the test on the same day, so you will need to register early if you want to get your preferred location. As with all standardized tests of this magnitude, you should research the test centers in advance. Given the choice, a small, out-of-the-way test center in a quiet location can offer the most stress-free and relaxed exam-taking environment.

The AAMC will mail you an admissions ticket several weeks before the test. You will not be allowed to enter the test site without this ticket, so put it somewhere safe. The AAMC's MCAT Web site has a wealth of specific information on the rules about taking the actual test. It's worth reviewing these to make sure you comply. The last thing you want to do is go through months of studying just to blow the test on a technicality.

About a week or two prior to the exam you should travel to the test site. Familiarize yourself with the location of the facility, how to get to the right room, and where the bathrooms are. If you're not a morning person, you should also start setting an alarm and get used to being awake and handling questions by the appointed start time of your upcoming exam. Beginning a week or so before the MCAT, several of us trained by getting up early and doing a bank of multiple-choice questions every day.

There are various rules and regulations about what you can and can't bring with you to the test. Most test centers will provide you with a locker or storage area in which to keep your personal belongings while you take the exam. It's worth packing a lunch and bringing some good high-energy snack foods with you for the break time. You'll be provided with everything you need to take the actual test, but you should *definitely* bring earplugs. You'll be in a large room with many stressed-out people, and the last thing you want is someone's sniffling or a nearby jackhammer breaking your concentration.

Finally, a word about the eleventh hour. Preparation for the MCAT is a marathon, not a sprint. Nothing you do the night before is going to change your score. The night before the test, get some exercise, eat a good meal, relax, and enjoy the evening off. Know that you're equipped with the knowledge and skills not just to take the test but actually to excel at it. Approach the test with calm confidence in the morning, and simply do the best you can.

WHATEVER THE SCORE, MAKE IT WORK FOR YOU

You should get your score results by mail within about sixty days. Before you open the results, make a promise to yourself that whatever they are, you will make them work for you. Performance on the test does vary year to year, so your MCAT score report will include statistical data to help you interpret your numbers. As mentioned previously, a basic rule of thumb is that a combined score of 30 will get you a solid consideration at a range of medical schools.

"When I reapplied for med school, I thankfully had to take the MCAT only once more," Deb notes. "I took my MCATs hoping I would either do really well or very poorly (naturally I prayed for 'really well'!). Unfortunately, I did absolutely average. I pondered whether or not to take the test again and decided to apply using those lackluster scores, figuring that if I didn't get an interview, I'd know I needed to take it again. Fortunately for me, I was invited to interview and then was accepted, so I escaped the pain of having to retake the MCATs. I think that my grades from college and high school were good enough to make my average MCAT scores acceptable."

So open your scores.

If you crushed the exam, congratulations—the MCAT has just become a major selling point of your application. If your scores are average, you'll be in the thick of the pack, so you'll have to let the other exceptional components of your application be your selling points. If you've underperformed, take stock. If your scores are only slightly below average, you'll want to consult your premed advisor for advice on how to proceed. If your scores are well below where they need to be to get into your chosen schools, drop back, assess what happened, punt, and plan on taking the test again.

If your strategy involves taking the test again, don't just repeat the experience. Make sure that next time around you allot yourself more time or adjust your study strategy to try new techniques and target the gaps in your substantive knowledge or procedural skills.

Remember, the road to medical school is a long one, sure to be paved with some ups and downs. Beating the MCAT is just one part of the marathon. If you have to take a second shot to overcome the MCAT, so be it. Your ultimate goal is admission to medical school, and the hallways of hospitals around the country are replete with doctors who needed a second chance to beat the MCAT.

PART TWO

Applying to
Medical School

CHAPTER 5

Crafting the Perfect Application

No man should part with his own individuality.
—WILLIAM ELLERY CHANNING

YOUR APPLICATION PROCESS officially begins the day you decide you want to go to medical school. This doesn't mean you should immediately sit down at the computer and tear your hair out trying to craft the perfect soul-searching personal statement. That can wait. But it is never too early to begin to understand the application process and the steps you'll need to take to secure a spot at the medical school of your choice. Starting early will not only make you aware of the requirements with sufficient time to respond to them, it will also foster your awareness of the attributes and gaps in your evolving application.

The medical-school application process is a chess game, and to play it well requires foresight, dedication, and strategy.

A QUICK OVERVIEW

Your first step in applying to med school is to familiarize yourself with the application process. Almost all medical schools use an initial, universal application produced and managed by the Association of American Medical Colleges (AAMC) and its American Medical College Application Service (AMCAS). You can review the list of AMCAS member medical schools using this universal application on the AMCAS Web site (www.amcas.org). This universal online application provides a common format for detailing all of your academic and extracurricular credentials and can be distributed to all the AM-CAS member schools of your choosing.

Individual schools then review this primary application and determine whether they wish to send you a secondary application. Thus, the first cut in the medical-school admissions game is whether or not you get a secondary application.

Each medical school crafts its own secondary application. Once your schools receive your secondary application (and, yes, an additional application fee), they decide whether to offer you an interview. This is the second cut in the process. Getting an interview puts you in the final round of applicants under consideration. After the interview, schools will admit, reject, or wait-list your application.

A timeline for the road ahead might look something like this:

Month	Activity
Summer after sophomore year (or one year prior to application)	• Start researching online Web sites and blogs to get the lay of the land and the latest tips and trends
August before junior year (or one year prior to application)	• Evaluate AMCAS requirements, identify personal strengths and weaknesses, and begin pulling materials together
September of junior year (or one year prior to application)	• Go to AAMC Web site and gather information about MCAT • Consult premed advisor for list of recommended resources • Develop personal MCAT study plan • Enroll in MCAT review course (if chosen)
December of junior year (or in year prior to application)	• Research test centers for MCAT administration on AAMC Web site • Identify and calendar MCAT registration date • Scope out various test centers and choose one
January of application year	• Register for MCAT

March of application year	• Meet with premed advisor to discuss application process • Solicit letters of recommendation from faculty
April of application year	• Take MCAT
May of application year	• Begin researching medical schools
June of application year	• Evaluate MCAT scores and begin finalizing application list • Begin drafting personal statement
July of application year	• Ensure that all faculty letters of recommendation have been received by college premed committee
August of senior/application year	• Upload completed AMCAS universal application
October of senior/application year	• All secondary applications complete
Fall/winter of senior/application year	• Interviews
Fall/winter of senior/application year	• Evaluate and rank acceptances • Keep in touch at schools where wait-listed
Winter of senior/application year	• Make a final decision and celebrate!

References and resources

Before we look at each of these application steps in detail, let's review some helpful resources. The AAMC Web site (www.aamc.org) is an excellent source of information. It provides a helpful array of tools and tables to help you to assess your strengths and weaknesses as a candidate (e.g., how does my undergraduate GPA stack up nationally, or at a particular school?) and also allows you to search and compare the attributes of every program in the country (e.g., how innovative is the curriculum at my favorite school?). Spend some time exploring this Web site and get familiar with it. As you march through the application process, you'll find it can be a very useful resource.

As noted a couple of chapters ago, the AAMC also produces a book called the *Medical School Admission Requirements (MSAR)*. This is a fairly comprehensive collection of the general requirements for medical school admission as well as all the individual, school-specific requirements, which will be very helpful to you in preparing your spreadsheet of individual application requirements and helping you stay organized. Purchase a copy, or at least consult a copy in any college library, career services office, or premed office. You can order your copy from the AAMC's Web site (www.aamc.org/medical schools.htm).

Finally, there is a wealth of information available to you on the Internet. Helpful hints, application tips, and information about various medical schools and their cultures can be found on e-mail subscription lists, and in chat rooms and blogs. One particularly helpful and stable site is the Student Doctor Network (www.student-doctor.net). Here, you will find a wide array of forums detailing everything from premed classes to choosing your residency. Web sites like these attract an online community of would-be physicians and provide a welcome opportunity to share ideas, ask questions, learn from each other's misadventures, or just plain commiserate.

The AMCAS universal application

As discussed above, the first step in the medical-school application process is the filing of the initial AMCAS universal application. A minority of schools do not subscribe to this system and rely only on their own applications for admission, but since you'll likely be applying to several schools, chances are very good you'll be filling out an AMCAS application.

The AMCAS universal application is comprised of the following sections:

- **Biographical Information:** All your basic identifying information, including your full legal name, your Social Security number, your contact information, and so forth.
- **Postsecondary Experiences:** Essentially your resume of extracurricular and postundergraduate activities. You're allowed

a maximum of fifteen, so you may have to condense your experiences into groups.

- **Scholastic Information:** You will need to obtain official transcripts from your undergrad and premed classes and painstakingly fill out the tables of classes and grades. The AAMC Web site will help you calculate a cumulative GPA. Be forewarned— the AAMC will compare the official transcripts from your schools with the data you enter into the course/grade tables, so don't exaggerate!
- **Standardized Tests:** Your MCAT scores will be automatically reported to the AAMC. If you wish to attach additional scores from other standardized tests, like the SAT, you can do so in this section.
- **Personal Statement/Essay:** A fairly open-ended one-page essay in which you are asked to explain your impetus for applying to medical school.

Spend some time on the AMCAS Web site getting the lay of the land. Register for a user name and password, and become familiar with the site, its tools, and its resources. Once you get a sense of the scope and type of information the primary application asks for, begin collecting the required materials. The goal here is not to start filling out the application immediately but to start gathering the necessary supporting materials and develop a sense of how your credentials stack up.

Make a file for your "Academic Record," and request the requisite number of official transcripts of your undergraduate work. If you completed your premed requirements after college, you'll need to provide a separate official transcript documenting those classes, and once again you will need to order the requisite number of copies in advance. Be forewarned: during the busy admissions season, it can take up to eight weeks to receive your official transcripts, so don't procrastinate on this task!

Your MCAT score reports also go in this file for safekeeping.

Make a separate file for "Honors, Awards, and Achievements," and get actual records of any awards and honors you've received so that when you describe them on your application you'll have specific descriptions and dates of the awards.

Finally, make a file of "Relevant Experiences," and list and summarize jobs, volunteer positions, and any and all experiences you've had that you feel contribute to your interest in medicine or to your general professional experience and persona. This can be everything from summer jobs as a camp counselor, in which you demonstrated leadership skills, to a bench-top research project you helped out on in college. When in doubt, be inclusive here.

> My postbac advisor said that a good application was a composite of three things: academic performance (GPA plus MCAT), community service, and research experience. Different schools place different weight on each of the three, but they form the foundation of an application. Any deficit in one (in my case, research experience) should be balanced by a stand-out performance in another. This set of advice is a simplistic but invaluable approach to putting together your application, and I cannot emphasize enough how many times I have seen people ignore this advice to their detriment. The important follow-through about this advice, however, is to realize that while it is your application that gets you the interview, it is the interview that gets you your acceptance.
>
> —Pete

A SELF-ASSESSMENT OF THE STRENGTH OF YOUR CREDENTIALS

Once you've surveyed the application landscape and gathered up the necessary information, it's time to take stock of where you are and determine how best to compile that information into a competitive application. There is, of course, no one perfect way to formulate a med-school application. There are, however, several key components that an admissions officer will be looking for. These include demonstrated scholastic aptitude, intellectual curiosity and drive, maturity and responsibility, integrity and the courage to act with that integrity, a desire to serve, and a sincere interest in health care or the practice of medicine.

Knowing this, do a general self-assessment and consider how your experiences will address these key points. If you find gaps or areas that need shoring up, doing this assessment early on will give you the opportunity to seek ways to round out your application. While you should never engage in an activity simply to pad your med-school application, it does make sense to identify gaps in your application and to find ways to optimize these areas.

Let's break out these components individually and examine what roles they play in your evolving application to medical school.

Scholastic fitness

Simply put, do you have the intellectual aptitude to meet the demands of the grueling med-school curriculum? Your application should accent academic experiences that required discipline, individualized research, or concentrated study and the mastering of difficult material. Do not limit yourself to experiences in the sciences. If you published your senior thesis examining the biblical implications of Melville's *Moby Dick,* that discussion goes here. Address any deficiencies head-on. Demonstrate that now, armed with maturity and a passion for medicine, you have what it takes to excel academically. If specific classes are a serious blot on your record, consider retaking one or two of them to prove you can handle the material.

Intellectual drive and curiosity

The premed curriculum has the capacity to turn people into drones. You go through the sequence of large premed courses as a well-orchestrated herd. Most of these classes leave little room for expressing individuality. Thus, it becomes important to demonstrate that you have an inherent intellectual curiosity and can pursue it independently.

Did you develop a research project with a faculty mentor and gain valuable hands-on research experience? Maybe you took time off to travel a part of the world to pursue a particular interest. Perhaps you spent some time teaching, writing, mastering an art, or playing music. Look to highlight specific occasions where you demonstrated a focused, individualized intellectual effort and discuss how the experience helped you grow.

Maturity and responsibility

Maturity and responsibility are obviously critical attributes of the successful med-school candidate. The role of physician is a weighty one. You will frequently be faced with major life-and-death decisions and trusted with the most sensitive details of people's lives. You must demonstrate not just that you've held positions of responsibility before but that you've carried off those responsibilities admirably. If your record is weak in this area, look for opportunities to get involved in leadership—take on a new responsibility at work, coach a team, spend some time teaching, or get involved with a community or professional organization or committee. As always, let your interests and passions drive you, but as you accomplish things, allow them to take their proper place in your application.

Integrity and ethical conduct

Ethical conduct as a scholar, a professional, and an individual is another essential quality for the physician. For most applicants, these attributes will be implied and need not be specifically demonstrated in your application. If you have had lapses or errors in judgment that will be revealed in your application, however, it is vitally important to address these circumstances head-on. Any sort of criminal record, especially one involving substance abuse, will be a matter of serious concern to admissions committees. You will need to prove that those issues are in your past and are no longer a problem for you. A letter of explanation accompanying your application is appropriate in these circumstances. If there are other personal or academic issues in your past, like other legal problems or expulsions for cheating, it would also be wise to discuss strategies for approaching these concerns with your premed advisor early on in the process.

Desire to serve

Medicine is an inherently service-oriented profession. At some fundamental level, all physicians are driven by a desire to help their patients, often setting aside their own needs to focus on their patients' needs. As such, demonstrating a dedication to public service is an important aspect of your application. If you haven't already done so, find a local hospital, rescue service, nursing home, or doctor's office and get involved. Travel to an underserved area and help out in a relief mission. Work at the local soup kitchen. Pick something you think you will enjoy. Try to develop a longer-term relationship with an organization that will enable you to develop relationships, demonstrate commitment, and develop some skills in a clinical setting.

Sincere interest in health care

Finally, a long-standing and profound interest in medicine is easy to demonstrate—if, that is, you've had a long-standing interest in medicine.

"Uh-oh," you say. "I just realized two months ago that this is what I want to do with my life—how am I supposed to pretend I've always wanted to be a doctor?"

You can't. And you shouldn't.

But you can reflect on the experiences you've had and define how they led you to your discovery of a passion for medicine. You can demonstrate that you've really explored and considered your decision to pursue medicine and that you are not acting on a whim. Spend time shadowing a physician, talk to other medical students about their experiences, or volunteer in a clinic, and then find some meaningful way to tie those experiences to your newfound interest in pursuing medicine. Remember that if your application lacks a clear, demonstrated interest in health care or medicine, you will need to convince an admissions committee, which is looking at thousands of other applicants who *can* demonstrate this commitment, that they should choose you.

CREATE A TIMELINE AND A MASTER TASK LIST

Staying organized and on top of your application requirements and deadlines is essential to the success of your application process. Applications are typically due in October or November of the year prior to matriculation. But there's a catch. Schools choose individually whether or not they wish to use the AMCAS universal application as an initial screen. Schools that do will likely await your finalized application to decide whether or not you qualify for a secondary application. Conversely, schools that do not use AMCAS as a screen may respond to the initial biographic data they receive from AMCAS (i.e., your name and address) by sending you a secondary application immediately, even before your AMCAS application is completed. This means two things. First, any and all material you put online for the universal application should be in final form. Second, you should get your AMCAS application up and running as early as possible to get your name into the applicant pool and facilitate your receipt of secondary applications early in the process.

A good benchmark is to try to get your AMCAS application on-line by mid-to-late August of your application year. This will give you time to review and complete your secondary applications and be competitive for the fall/winter interview season. The longer you wait, the bigger the applicant pool and the stiffer the competition.

So, let's work backward from that date.

About a year prior to that, you should begin to scrutinize the AMCAS application and gather your materials. This means if you're still an undergraduate, you should begin the preliminaries of your med-school application process in the fall of junior year. Spend the fall and winter of your junior year doing a realistic self-assessment, listing and examining your application strengths and weakness, and developing a plan to smooth the edges and fill in the gaps. Make sure you meet the fall deadlines for application to the April MCAT if you haven't already taken it (refer to chapter 4 for details about the MCAT). In early spring, meet with your premed advisor about your application. By midspring start asking for your letters of recommendation. By June you should begin drafting your personal statement for the AMCAS application. All your letters of recommendation should be received by your college's premed committee by the end of July, and you should be actively creating your application online. Aim to complete your AMCAS application by mid-to-late August. The deadline is October 1.

Let's look more closely at each of these application milestones.

Getting organized

In the fall prior to your intended application season, you should start getting organized. Peruse the AAMC and AMCAS Web sites. Download the application materials and get familiar with them. Complete the self-assessment as outlined above, and make a list of the areas where you feel strongest and the areas where you feel your application could use some shoring up. Actively seek opportunities and experiences that can address these needs. Starting early gives you a full year to remedy any obvious weaknesses.

How to use your premed advisor

The next step is to meet with your premed advisor. If you're doing your premed studies as a postbac, you may elect to use your advisor at your original undergraduate institution or the advisor at the school where you've done your most recent course work. Pick the person who will have the most insight into your current academic abilities and who is likely to carry the most weight with an admissions committee.

Either way, in March of your application year, take your folders of application materials with you and sit down with your advisor to discuss your application. Lay out your record and candidly discuss your strengths and weaknesses. Develop a plan to remedy any remaining identified deficiencies. Discuss which of your experiences stand out and merit emphasis in your application. Most important, ask for a letter of recommendation from your premed advisor. While you may barely know this person, and thus a letter from him or her may seem to carry limited value, most schools either look for or require a letter from the premed advisor or committee at your college or university. While the letter may not provide the most intimate, personal spin on your candidacy, the advisor or committee will be able to objectively comment on your performance in your premed class work relative to your peers.

The categorical rank your premed advisor gives to your application will provide admissions committees with a somewhat objective measure of your undergrad and premed successes. In addition, most premed advisors or committees require that all your letters of recommendation be sent directly to them so that they can review and summarize your other recommenders' comments in their letter. They then collate the stack of letters, lead with their own letter, and send the package off to your selected schools.

Given the influence that your premed advisor will have in the process, the importance of getting to know this person on a personal level cannot be overstated. People generally go the extra mile to help people they *know* and *like*. In the highly competitive process of med-school admissions, every incremental advantage helps . . . and this is one that a lot of applicants will overlook.

Don't be one of them.

Spring of your junior year is also a good time to begin researching which schools you should apply to. In this age of online resources, this task has never been easier. Use the AAMC Web site and the various med-school home pages to evaluate schools, learn which schools use which teaching formats, and generate ideas about which schools interest you. During your meeting with your premed advisor, ask for some advice on schools you should consider, given your academic record and interests. In many cases, your premed advisor will have particular insight about, and may recommend, specific schools that look favorably on graduates from your undergraduate institution.

Start broadly, gradually narrowing your search and shortening your list as you receive feedback from your premed advisor and learn more about what schools offer.

Choosing which medical schools to apply to will be an ongoing process over the next six months or so, so don't feel that you need to make any final decisions today. (Chapter 6 covers this process in detail.) Gather information and advice from a broad range of sources. Remember that family, friends, mentors, and your premed advisor will all weigh in, but ultimately, the decision about where to apply is yours to make.

Take the MCAT in the spring

As mentioned previously, it is optimal to take the MCAT at the April administration of your junior year, or, if you are applying postbac, in the April prior to application season. Ideally, you will have just completed your premed studies and will be primed to perform on the test. By taking the test in April, you will ensure that you have your scores back in June—well before your applications are due, which will give you more insight into your strength as a candidate and more opportunities to hone your strategy.

Soliciting letters of recommendation

By midspring of your application year, your file should really be starting to take shape. The next step is soliciting your letters of recommendation. Most schools require at least three letters, two of which should be from science faculty at your undergraduate or premed institutions. Typically, you will solicit four to six letters and ask the writers to send them directly to your premed committee. As discussed above, the committee will, in turn, review the letters and your academic record and then write a cover letter of recommendation. They will then send all the letters directly to the schools you're applying to. If your school does not provide a premed committee or if you have been out of school for some time, you may elect to hire a commercial service such as Interfolio (www.interfolio.com) to handle your letters of recommendation for you. For a fee, such companies will collect your individual letters of recommendation and send them to specific schools by specific dates. This spares your letter writers from the need to send individual letters to each school you apply to.

The key to getting a good letter is identifying someone who knows you personally, can speak to the quality of your work and work ethic, and can address your fitness to be a medical student. In general, letters from celebrity figures like senators, governors, or hospital CEOs do not carry much weight with admissions committees unless the celebrity recommender can actually comment substantially about your candidacy. Similarly, letters from family members or direct personal friends without a professional tie are of limited value. Further, professors who are just looking at your resume and don't know you personally rarely write convincing letters.

"But wait a minute," you say. "The premed courses at my school all had several hundred students in them! How was the professor supposed to get to know me personally?"

We're glad you asked that.

If you find yourself needing letters from faculty who don't know you, you'll need to help them *get* to know you! Schedule appointments with those professors during their office hours. Drop off a copy of your resume and a one- or two-page prose "bio sheet" in advance to help highlight who you are. At the meeting, discuss your resume, your life experiences, and your broader goals and intentions with them. Help them get to know you as a person so they can illuminate your recommendation with some personal observations.

"When I was a premed student, I shadowed my own primary-care doctor every Tuesday morning for about two months," one mentor explained. "I would meet her at the hospital, do rounds, and then spend a few hours in her office seeing patients. It was an extraordinary experience for me, but it also helped her get to know me better and, thus, to write me a more meaningful recommendation."

"I used a potpourri approach for my letters," Pete notes. "My first and strongest letter was from a physician mentor who knew me very well personally and professionally. My graduate school advisor wrote one for me, as did my employer in Oakland. My premed advisor from my postbac program did a phenomenal job in collecting comments and putting together a letter on my behalf. I do recommend getting a variety of people to write for you, and making sure they know you well is certainly the most important piece."

"I think getting letters from professors is good, but I think it is best to get letters from people who know you well," Carolyn says. "I felt okay about getting a letter from a TA, because I felt he had a good grasp of my potential."

Asking for letters of recommendation should not be an uncomfortable task. Most of the people you will ask have had to write many such letters and are accustomed to such requests. Be forthright and polite, and go to them at least eight weeks in advance of the date you need the letters. Be clear about the deadlines, and also give them an out by explaining that you need a strong endorsement of your candidacy for medical school, and if they don't think they can provide one, they should decline. If you request a letter from someone and find them waffling, politely withdraw your request and move on to someone else on your list. The last thing you want is a lukewarm recommendation.

Be sure to provide each of your recommenders with the appropriate forms, and stamped envelopes addressed to the premed committee or wherever you want the letter sent. Write your full name on the inside flap of the envelope to ensure that the professor's assistant puts the right letters in the right envelopes. While you technically have the right to review all letters written on your behalf, it is best to waive this right. Most admissions directors put more stock in candid letters and are wary of students that feel they need to see their letters of recommendation. In many cases, your recommenders will provide you with a courtesy copy of their letters anyway.

Do not underestimate the impact that a strong letter of recommendation can have on your application. A comprehensive letter from a solid source who knows you well can speak volumes about your integrity and the quality of your work. "My recommendations and my essay were the highlights of my application," Adam notes. "They helped compensate for some middle-of-the-road numbers in terms of grades and scores. People choosing future doctors know that your success in medicine is not directly related to your ability to test well; rather, it is determined by your ability to relate to people and earn their trust. This has become increasingly apparent throughout my residency."

Crafting the perfect personal statement

You should begin working on your personal statement no later than the beginning of June of your application year. For most people, this is the most difficult component of the application process.

"As with most things of this nature, I agonized over my essay," Deb recalls. "I really wanted to come up with something original, but in the end took the age-old approach of 'why I want to go to medical school.' My essay was not very original, but it allowed me to discuss my experiences and how they led me to medical school."

At its best, a personal statement can make your application truly stand out and will make the admissions reader say, "Wow, I've got to meet this person." At its worst, an essay that is rife with errors, poorly constructed, arrogant, or offensive can immediately and utterly derail your candidacy. Your personal statement should, at the very least, give an admissions committee a window into your life and a good sample of your writing and communications skills.

"My essay was pure self-promotion," Pete says. "I knew as an older student with multiple former careers (all of which happened to be tropical), as well as an acceptable but hardly exemplary undergraduate performance, I had to spin my unique background into a statement showing what positive impacts those experiences had on my life and on my decision to go into medicine. I would advise choosing a topic that sets you apart from the mob of students applying for each spot, without coming across as too esoteric."

So how do you go about writing an effective personal statement? Like everything else in this process, start early, think creatively, and keep at it. In the end, the best personal statement is one that is sincere and demonstrates something about you and your desire to be a doctor. Reflect on your experiences and achievements and on the decision-making process you've experienced to this point. See if you can tease out themes or experiences that were especially formative or unique.

"I wrote about how I made the decision to go to medical school specifically because it wasn't an obvious trend in the rest of my biography," Ben explains. "As such, I cited specific examples of events that contributed to my thinking process."

Once you have settled on your subject matter, start putting together a first draft. Your essay should ultimately be about one thousand words in length. It should have a clear and logical structure, harkening back to the standard five-paragraph essay (an intro, three main points, and a conclusion) from eighth-grade English class. Remember that admissions directors read thousands of these statements each year, so do your best to make yours clear, readable, and interesting. While creativity is absolutely a plus, bizarre, outlandish, or offensive material is a definite no-no. Find someone who is a good editor and get them to read your drafts. As you get closer to a final edit, solicit reactions from a wider audience. Capitalize on the opportunity to explain who you are as a person. Make sure you have anyone and everyone look for errors, and make the message come alive on the page.

Putting it all together

It's now late summer of your application year. You've met with your premed advisor, solicited your letters of recommendation, completed the MCAT, sought additional clinical experience, and finalized your course work. Your personal statement is in final form.

Now it's time to put it all together.

This may seem like the easiest part, and in many ways it is. However, it's also one of the more intricate and important things to be done. Just as you spent hours perfecting your personal statement, so you should devote serious attention to making your application perfect. Start by uploading all of your relevant scholastic and work experience. Review your uploaded transcripts and make sure they reflect your most up-to-date work. Describe your extracurricular activities and experiences using active, vibrant verbs, and craft your descriptions of them to address the overall objectives presented in the beginning of this section. Carefully upload your personal statement. Once you have all the information in the application, print it out and review it in detail. Make sure it is properly formatted to look good on the printed page, since the admissions committees will typically print and read it in hard copy. Get a trusted editor to review it for you one final time. The hard-copy pages in front of you will be your first opportunity to shine for the admissions committee, and first impressions are lasting ones. When you can't stand looking at the thing one second longer, look it over one more time and submit it.

Now it's time to move on to choosing your schools.

CHAPTER 6

Choosing Your School

The wise man bridges the gap by laying out the path by means of which he can get from where he is to where he wants to go.
—J. P. MORGAN

WITH YOUR INITIAL AMCAS application uploaded and online, you're ready to pick your schools. As with all of your previous application decisions, this is one you'll want to linger over and consider carefully.

RESEARCH RESOURCES

The first step in choosing a school is learning about the options. Again, your best friend here will be the Internet, and specifically the AAMC Web site (www.aamc.org). It has a complete listing of all 125 accredited allopathic medical schools in the United States as well as the seventeen accredited Canadian schools. The site also features various tools to compare and contrast different schools based on location, curricular innovation, admissions statistics, and the like. The admissions contacts page contains links to each medical school's home page, allowing you to delve further into the schools you're interested in. Similar information is available on The American Association of Colleges of Osteopathic Medicine's (AACOM) Web site (www.aacom.org) for the twenty accreditied D.O. schools in the United States.

Your premed advisor will be another useful source of informational guidance. He or she is specifically tasked with helping you find a seat at the best possible medical school for your needs and preferences. Your premed advisor should also be clued in to the very latest trends and issues in medical education and to the current status of the various programs across the country. When you meet with your advisor in the spring of your application year, have at least a tentative list of schools to discuss. This discussion will help you assess how realistic you've been in your selection of schools and help your advisor understand what criteria you're using to select your schools. This early calibration will be a real asset in helping to ensure the success of your admissions process.

Friends, colleagues, and mentors in medicine or in medical education may provide additional insights. Be cautious in relying too heavily on this information, though, since it may reflect personal biases or be out of date.

Many people also use the *U.S. News & World Report* annual ranking of medical schools. While these rankings are widely consulted and often quoted in the popular media, the reality is that the criteria they use to rank the top medical schools may have little to do with the factors you are most concerned about. The AAMC Web site features an interesting treatment of this issue, which you should review. While all of your mentors admit to consulting the *U.S. News & World Report* rankings when developing their lists of preferred schools, most used it only as a launching pad to further research, and none cited it as the determining factor in their ultimate choice of which school to attend.

Finally, before you start casting your net, it's a good idea to start closest to home. Your state school is not only almost always your cheapest option, it also tends to be your most certain option. Although not all states have their own state medical school, the ones that don't almost always have an affiliated school in a neighboring state. You should almost certainly submit an application to this state school, even if it's not a top choice for you. Spend some time evaluating this program, perusing its Web site, and if possible visiting the campus and talking to students. Learn all you can about its program so that as you begin to research other schools you have a baseline against which to compare. This initial effort will help you to hone your investigative skills and develop an intelligent wish list for your ideal program.

Finalizing Your List and Weighing Your Decision

Now that you've surveyed the field and gotten a sense of what's out there, the next question is: how do you determine which program is best for you? As you begin this process you may be saying to yourself, "I don't care where I go, I just want to get in somewhere." Or you may be saying, "I have to go to Yale." But spend some time considering the primary differentiators likely to affect your school decision—location, curriculum, reputation, and cost—and develop your list accordingly.

Location

Location is the first way most people start narrowing their list. As mentioned, your state or state-affiliated school usually offers you the twin advantages of lower cost and increased likelihood of admission. It also offers you the opportunity to attend school in an area you already know and stay near family and friends—resources you may need to draw on during the stressful times in medical school. Location may also be a factor if you have a spouse or significant other who is tied to a specific job or industry that has geographic constraints.

As you consider schools outside your geographic location, think about places you'd like to live and work for four or more years. Is the school in a big city or a small town? What activities outside of school are available there? How easy is it to travel to and from the school? What is the ethnic mix in the area? Where do most people who attend the school come from? What is the medical community like in the area where the school is located? What is the climate like? Answer as many of these types of questions as you can, then try to pare down the list of 125 schools accordingly.

"Location was very important for me," Kate explains. "I wanted to stay in the New England area. My free time was precious, and I did not want to have to spend time traveling back to New England. I wanted to be close to family and friends for support."

"When I decided to reapply, I applied to only one school—the University of Colorado," Deb adds. "I had been in Denver since college and really enjoyed my life in this locale. All of my friends were here. I was in a serious relationship with my future husband, Steve, who had all of his friends and a great job here in Denver. We loved the mountains, skiing, the weather—we just didn't want to move. We decided that I would apply to CU only and see how things went. If I didn't get in, the next year I would expand my list. Looking back now, if I hadn't gotten in, I probably would have just kept reapplying to CU. Location was huge!"

Curriculum

The next major differentiator will likely be curriculum. This is a vitally important attribute to consider, yet a difficult one to evaluate from the outside. As discussed in chapter 2, the last decade has seen radical innovations in the way medical school curricula are constructed and evaluated. At many schools, the traditional curriculum, with monolithic blocks of two years of basic sciences followed by two years of clinical rotations, is gone. Many med schools have recognized that students need and desperately want an integrated curriculum in which the clinical relevance of material is emphasized, and in which they have the opportunity to develop a foundation of medical knowledge and the nascient clinical skills simultaneously.

Unfortunately, such innovation has also led to a dizzying array of options that can be bewildering to the would-be med student. Again, the AAMC Web site is helpful here, in that it can help you establish some common themes and marked differences to help you better compare and contrast among and between programs. Only you can determine what combination of pure science, integrated clinical studies, and small-group learning is best for your learning style. Think about how you learn and interact with others, and then aim for the schools whose curriculum has an almost visceral appeal.

Reputation

Everyone wants to go to the best med school in the country. The only problem is, no one is certain what school that is.

What does "number 1" mean?

Who is doing the judging?

What criteria are they using, and do those criteria match your interests?

The truth is there's no truly objective ranking of schools available. The most popular ranking, clearly, is the annual *U.S. News &*

World Report list. However, the criteria that they use may have limited relevance to the criteria that matter most to you.

So should reputation really matter at all, then?

The answer to that question is that it probably only matters in the extremes. If you graduate from one of the med schools that is particularly well known and respected (fairly or not), doing so will likely have a favorable impact on your residency application and future career direction. Similarly, if you graduate from a bottom-tier or off-shore medical school, this may make your match and subsequent career path considerably more challenging. Outside these extremes, the individual merits of your performance, your recommendations, and your application coming out of medical school will be the metric by which you are judged. So, in general, the reputation of the school you attend will have only a moderate impact on your residency or career.

"Doing well in medical school is vastly more important than where you go to medical school," Adam explains. "I am currently a resident at Johns Hopkins and have had the opportunity to work with many of the current medical students here. Their performance on the wards seems to be the single most important factor in where they go for residency. My fellow residents are from medical schools all over the country, and which school they attended has not been a strong differentiator of performance."

In assessing the relative reputations of the various schools on your list, you should also consult your premed advisor, who will, no doubt, provide additional perspective on the med-school market and current trends and challenges. Solicit your advisor's top ten list of schools along with his explanations for these choices, and if there's a particular specialty that you think you might be interested in pursuing, ask your advisor and practitioners in that field for their lists of top schools in that discipline. Most schools are very strong in some areas and weak in others, so finding a school that has demonstrated excellence in the areas of your greatest interest is a good approach to take.

Cost

Finally, you should consider cost in your school selection criteria, though you should never let cost dissuade you from considering any given school. There are numerous mechanisms to fund your entry to even the most expensive private medical schools, and you will ultimately be able to manage whatever debt load you undertake. It is also true, however, that educational debt can be a significant burden and may have a significant impact on your life after residency. In 2006, the average debt load for graduating medical students was approximately $114,000. That isn't chump change, and it doesn't include other short-term debt like credit cards and car payments, which average an additional $22,000. To put these numbers in perspective, if you graduated today with that debt load and consolidated your loans to a single thirty-year amortized loan, your monthly payment would be on the order of $600 to $1,000 per month, depending on interest rates. If your debt load is $250,000 because you are also carrying undergraduate debt, your monthly payment could be twice that amount. Given that when you finally start your practice you will likely have a mortgage payment, and perhaps a family to support, the numbers add up fast.

"Location was extremely important to me in the initial screening," Pete explains. "Cost initially was not a strong consideration, but when the acceptances were in and the decision had to be made, it became more important. Cost is something I would stress extremely heavily to potential applicants, and it's something that is not emphasized enough in premed discussions. In short, survey after survey shows that the amount of debt directly influences how medical students choose their specialty. An inexpensive education buys you the freedom to pursue the path you want to take."

So how should you use cost considerations in school selection? First, do a self-assessment of your current financial status. Do you have significant undergraduate debt that will require repayment? Do you have outstanding credit card debt? Do you own your own home or have other major investments?

Next, consider the lifestyle choices you anticipate making postgraduation. Are you determined to live in an expensive city, to own your own boat or a second home? Are you hoping to practice rurally or in an underserved area? Are you a member of the armed forces, or interested in making a commitment for service? All these are factors that may have a significant impact on your earning potential.

Recognize that if you're determined to attend a school with very high tuition, you may have to make sacrifices on the other side to manage your debt load. Those sacrifices might be a leaner lifestyle for a while, a period of service in an underserved area or to the armed forces in exchange for debt relief, or a need to pursue a higher-paying specialty to facilitate your loan repayment.

"In retrospect, I should have thought more about cost," Ben reflects. "Almost all schools train you well or they wouldn't be accredited. Being saddled with two hundred thousand dollars in debt, though, is another thing entirely."

Making your list and checking it twice

So you've done your research and successfully winnowed your list of potential schools down to your top choices. For some, there may be only a handful of schools that meet your criteria (or possibly just one school if family or other obligations force you to stay in your immediate area). For others, this refined list may still be quite long. In the end there's no magic number of schools you should apply to. While a shotgun approach of applying to every school you can find may optimize your exposure, it certainly won't guarantee acceptance. Conversely, having your heart set on a single institution and applying solely there may prove foolhardy—unless you're willing to wait and continue reapplying until you eventually get in. As with most things, moderation is your best bet.

In 2005, the average med-school applicant applied to eleven schools, and the old adage from your undergrad days to apply to a three-tiered mix of schools carries over to medical school as well. Typically this would be a mix of two to three safety schools where your MCAT score and undergraduate GPA make you a promising candidate (including your in-state school), several midrange schools where your GPA and MCAT scores indicate that you should be a solid competitor, and a group of reach schools where you hope some aspect of your application will strike a chord with someone and make the stars align for you.

Again, the specific forces driving your candidacy will shape your application list, so this is just a general rule of thumb. Your premed advisor should be able to help you tailor your application list to your specific needs. The AAMC application Web site is set up so that you pay $160 for the first school and $30 for each additional school. Be sure you apply only to schools you would actually go to if you were accepted!

CHAPTER 7

Finalizing Your AMCAS Application and Completing Your Secondaries

Once more unto the breach.
—WILLIAM SHAKESPEARE

ONCE YOU PAY the fee correlating to your school selection, AM-CAS will send your completed application dossier to each of the schools you selected. Any changes you make to the AMCAS application from this point forward will be received by your target schools as change-updates. In other words, finding a series of errors in your original submission and sending a bunch of changes along will not reflect well on your ability to handle precision work, so make sure it is complete and *perfect* before you submit it.

Shortly after you submit your AMCAS application, contact each of the schools on your final list and make sure they show your admissions file as complete. While AMCAS does a good job handling the administrative burden posed by this process, mistakes do happen. Take no chances—follow up with every school on your list.

SECONDARY APPLICATIONS

With your AMCAS application filed, and all schools reporting your file as complete, the waiting game truly begins. When and how will the secondaries arrive? Before you begin holding a vigil at the mailbox, remember that we're living in the electronic era. These days, your first news will likely come by e-mail, followed by a packet in the mail.

In an ideal world, medical schools would review your primary AMCAS application, weigh your credentials against your peers', and offer secondary applications only to the students they feel are qualified for admission. One would also hope that their secondary application would expound on the primary application, giving you the opportunity to highlight your unique characteristics or comment on why you're interested in that particular school. In such a world, by completing your secondary application and paying your second application fee, you could justifiably feel like you were in the game.

Unfortunately, it doesn't always work that way. Many schools see the secondary application as a financial turnstile and will send out secondaries to *anyone* who submits a primary application. Worse still, many of the secondaries are just reformatted versions of the information on the primary application, and some schools will *still* apply some objective screening criteria that they could have derived from the primary application.

In other words, receiving a secondary application from a school does not necessarily mean that you are in the ball game. You may be looking at hours and hours to perfect a whole new redundant application, and paying another $40–$100 per application, *only to be rejected outright because you don't meet a school's threshold screening criteria, which they could have derived from your AMCAS universal application.*

Frustrating, isn't it?

Unfortunately, there's no way around this one, and no good way to say which schools employ these methods, since, understandably, med schools tend to be fairly tight-lipped about how their individual admissions systems work—particularly when the system is financially advantageous.

There is tremendous variability in the format of secondary applications. Nonetheless, there are still a few salient points to keep in mind.

First, these applications will likely be scrutinized even more closely than your primary application, so attention to detail remains paramount. Second, where possible, use every opportunity to *expand* on the content from your primary application instead of merely repeating it. You want to offer the admissions committee as much useful information about yourself as you can. In fact, you should answer every question on a secondary application completely—never leave blanks on the assumption that the admissions committee can get the information from your primary application. Never write "See Attached Resume" as an answer, as doing so is an invitation to an over-worked admissions officer to move on *without* doing so.

Allow a significant amount of time to complete your secondaries. Many schools place a deadline on your secondary response, often giving you as little as two weeks to return the application. When several secondaries with tight deadlines arrive at the same time, the pressure can mount. Furthermore, if you're a senior in college at this point, this process usually heats up just as the fall semester is getting under way.

Take your time, stay organized, and ensure quality control. Your secondaries are the key to the next stage of the process. Be sure they represent your very best work.

With your secondaries complete, it is time to play the waiting game again. You must now sit back and hope that the various med-school admissions committees look favorably upon your hard work.

CHAPTER 8

How to Ace Your Med-School Interviews

A word in earnest is as good as a speech.
—CHARLES DICKENS

HOPEFULLY THE LONG days of waiting with bated breath for an e-mail or the mailman have brought dividends.

The news, of course, will not always be good. Few people will get interviews everywhere they apply, and a substantial number of students will be rejected everywhere on their first attempt. Don't panic, and don't feel bad if this is you. According to the AAMC, in 2004, there were 35,735 applicants, 27,189 of whom were first-time applicants (76 percent). There were 17,662 acceptance offers made, which translates into a 49 percent acceptance rate. Roughly half of all applicants got accepted nowhere, and roughly half of those went on to reapply in 2005.

We hope you'll land a seat at the school of your choice on your first attempt, and this chapter teaches you how to campaign in person for that offer of admission. If you're contemplating your first interview, read ahead for advice on how to excel in this next and critical phase of your application process. If you've failed to secure any interviews, however, don't despair. Recognize that you're actually in the majority of applicants, and skip ahead to the next chapter for advice about how to proceed.

HOW TO CHOOSE AND PRIORITIZE YOUR INTERVIEWS

The first issue to address is how to manage multiple interviews spread all over the country. Obviously, this is a pleasant problem to have, though if you've applied to a range of schools with disparate geography, the financial implications of crisscrossing the country and putting yourself up in hotels for a dozen interviews is significant.

Be very cautious, however, in rejecting any offer to interview.

Take all the interviews you can get, and become more selective only as you develop increasing perspective about the market, your strength as a candidate, or if your desires to attend a school have diminished.

Wherever possible, try to group your interviews by region and date so that you can minimize the number of trips you have to take. If you've been offered an interview at one or more med schools that you applied to in a given geographic region, call the admissions offices of the other schools you applied to in that region and try some guerilla marketing tactics. *Politely* and *humbly* explain to an admissions officer that you are going to be in the region interviewing at one or more schools, that you remain very interested in that school, and you would love the opportunity to interview on the same trip, if possible. Doing this serves to reinforce your interest in the school, forces the admissions director to review your application again, and also puts subtle pressure on the school to consider you in a more favorable light since other, potentially competitive schools in the same region thought you were qualified enough to warrant an interview.

One caveat to this approach:

Never, never, *ever* misrepresent your status at other schools. If you don't actually have any other interviews in the region on those dates, don't say you do. The world of med-school admissions is a small one, and admissions directors do talk, particularly on a regional level. There's no faster way to destroy your candidacy to medical school than lying to an admissions director.

Some schools interview a set number of candidates and will make their final acceptance decisions only at the very end of the season after all interviews are over. At these schools, the timing of your interviews is not that significant. Other schools, however, use a rolling-admissions system in which the admissions staff meets periodically to decide which of the candidates they've seen thus far should be offered admission. For schools that offer rolling admission, schedule your interviews as early as possible in the admissions season, when the committee has a full class to fill and has seen fewer candidates.

Preparing for Your Interviews

While it may feel like you are the one on the hot seat during an interview, the truth is that the best interviews are really two-way conversations. Remember that even though it's a seller's market, the interview is not just an opportunity for the school to evaluate you as a candidate for admission. It's also an opportunity for you to evaluate what the school has to offer for your education. Empower yourself as a consumer to ask tough questions and discover the relative strengths and weaknesses of the programs you apply to. Naturally, your inquiries should always be respectful. Asking thoughtful, insightful, and comparative questions specific to the program, however, shows that you are a confident and educated consumer who has done your homework.

"Be polite and courteous to everyone," Adam counsels. "I saw a few applicants shoot themselves in the foot by being rude or short with secretaries in the admissions office. Respect your interviewers whether they are medical students or faculty—both votes are weighted equally when the committee makes its final decision."

Structure of the interview

Most med-school interviews are structured similarly. You meet in the morning with the admissions director and all the other candidates interviewing that day. There is typically a short presentation by the admissions director welcoming you and giving specifics about the program. After this, you'll go on a campus tour, usually given by a senior med student. This is a good opportunity to get a student's perspective on the campus and student life, as well as current campus issues.

When the tour is over, you will be assigned a sequence of interviews. Most interviews last about thirty minutes, are typically with a subset of the admissions committee, and can include clinical faculty, research faculty, and upper-level students. A few schools use a panel interview, in which you'll sit in front of three or four interviewers at the same time. After your interviews, some schools will ask you to complete a brief writing exercise. This is often a brief ethics case, where you will be expected to handwrite a single-page response. This is an opportunity for the school to evaluate how you think on your feet and compose and organize your thoughts on paper. There may be some closing remarks from the admissions director, and then you'll be on your way, mentally and physically exhausted, back to the hotel to pack up and hopefully do it all again somewhere else in a day or two.

So how do you go about preparing for this experience?

The first step in your preparation, as usual, is research. Start with the school's Web site. Garner all the information you can about the current first-year class, curricular structure, clinical rotations, and extracurricular activities. Look for information on school news, current projects, or future plans. Look up the local newspaper on the Internet and do a quick search to see if the school has been in the news lately.

Many schools also offer on-campus admissions sessions prior to interview season. If it's a local school, or a school that is high on your list, try to attend one of these sessions. If you know someone at the school, buy them a cup of coffee and solicit an insider's view of the advantages and the shortcomings of the program.

Gathering this information needn't be an exhaustive, time-consuming project. You're just looking to collect some good basic information. Summarize your findings in a list of topics to be discussed during your interview. Consider categorizing your list into aspects of the school that you especially like, areas you would like clarification about, and areas that concern you. Finally, make a list of three or four questions that you can draw on in a pinch if there's a lag or an awkward pause in any of your conversations. These might include questions like "What's on the horizon for the school that you're excited about?" or "If you could change two things about your program, what would they be?"

"Do your homework on the school you are applying to by reading their brochures and handouts," Pete suggests. "If you get a list of interviewers, do a quick Internet search on them just so you know what their basic interests are."

While you must remember that you're presenting yourself to the school, interviewers are people, too, and they'll often note your knowledge of their program with interest.

Practicing your interview

Once you've completed your research, it's time to perfect your interviewing skills. For some, interviewing is a natural, comfortable task. For others it is a white-knuckled, anxiety-provoking terror session. If you fall into the latter group, interviewing may never be fun for you, but a little practice will help you to reduce your anxiety and project yourself more competently and more effectively.

The questions you encounter in an interview will vary widely. There are, however, some common questions that seem to pop up again and again. It's worth rehearsing these subjects to gain comfort in discussing them, or versions of them, at the drop of a hat. Reread your application again and try to tie specifics to the basic themes. Here are some of the most common questions to stimulate your thinking:

- Why do you want to go to medical school? Why our medical school?
- What are your particular strengths and weaknesses?
- What adjectives would you use to describe yourself?
- When did you decide you wanted to become a doctor?
- What experiences were especially formative in your decision to become a doctor?
- What unique skills or attributes do you believe you would bring to the school?
- In your personal statement you mentioned . . . Tell me more about that.

If you've already experienced a professional job interview at some point in your life, the experience should be familiar. The interview will begin with some standard pleasantries, followed by some comments about your application. Resist the urge to apologize for or react defensively about any areas of weakness, even if they are pointed out to you. Instead, offer a matter-of-fact explanation, and then explain how the experience surrounding that weakness helped you grow, or what you gained from it. Endeavor to demonstrate a passion for your subject and your experiences. A little self-deprecating humor, if well chosen, can help break the ice, project confidence, and make everyone more comfortable with each other. Try to be responsive to the questions asked of you, but don't do so by merely regurgitating the material in your application. Try to add detail or to summarize your experiences in a new way. Attempt to tie the questions you're asked to your fitness as a med-student candidate or your hopes for your career as a physician. Have confidence in yourself, and try to be as relaxed and as natural as possible.

In the next phase of the interview, your interviewer will typically ask if you have any questions. This is your opportunity to do two things. First, by asking some questions specific to the school and to their educational program, you can demonstrate a sincere interest in the particular program and that you are an informed consumer who has done your homework. Second, it's an opportunity for you to gauge their responses and use those responses to better assess how attractive the program and the school are to you. Don't be afraid to ask the tough questions, but do so in a way that invites explanation and avoids confrontation or an overt display of skepticism on your part. Open-ended questions like, "What do you feel is the greatest strength and greatest weakness in your program?" are always good to get the conversation going. Be sure to follow up on your inter-viewer's response, though, to avoid the appearance of asking canned questions. Your goal should be an engaging conversation, not a rote exchange of lists.

Finally, a few schools may throw you a real curveball question. These questions are highly variable and are meant to assess your abil-ity to think on your feet and be creative. Some questions are just odd ("If you were an animal, what animal would you be and why?" or, "What's the most dastardly thing you've ever done?"). You simply can't prepare for these questions, and you shouldn't get too anxious over them. A polite chuckle, a moment or two of reflection, and the best response that comes to mind is usually appropriate . . . and a bit of well-chosen humor is always welcome. Don't fear a moment or two of silence in an interview—these moments are okay, and your ability to allow them to occur projects confidence and maturity.

Don't make yourself crazy preparing for or scripting your inter-view responses. Just try to get to a place where you are comfortable with a range of topics and potential questions, and where you are in-timately familiar with your application materials and can discuss any aspect of them with ease. In the end, interviewing is simply a skill some people excel at and others find extremely challenging. If you're in the former category, the interview can be your chance to shine and to really make your application come alive. If you're in the latter category, your job in the interview is to simply assert yourself professionally and let your strengths shine elsewhere.

Conquering your nerves

Let's face it. It is almost impossible not to be nervous on interview day. You've done a tremendous amount of work to get to this point, and it's hard not to feel like your entire future may be riding on the next few hours. Your strongest weapon against the encroachment of anxiety is a sense of confidence tempered with humility.

"I tried to prepare answers to questions I was fairly certain I would be asked and then practiced my delivery," Chris recalls. "I found the hardest part of interviewing was not coming up with the answers but controlling my nervous energy."

"My advice is to be extremely confident in yourself as a person and an applicant, while at the same time being respectful and humble in the face of requesting admittance to the world of medicine," Pete suggests. "It sounds trite, but to find that balance is to come across as the perfect candidate."

TOP TEN INTERVIEW DOS AND DON'TS

1. Do dress professionally and conservatively. Yes, that means a suit.
2. Don't use profane language, and avoid being bigoted or biased.
3. Do show up fifteen minutes early on interview day. Never, never, ever be late.
4. Don't respond angrily or provoke confrontation, no matter what the question.
5. Do look people in the eye, speak clearly and with confidence, and shake hands firmly. Politely but unapologetically thank people for their time and their consideration of your candidacy.
6. Don't slouch, appear overly casual or disinterested, or name drop.
7. Do ask open-ended questions and attempt to get your interviewer to talk about his or her experiences as well.
8. Don't wear heavy perfume or colognes, excessive or gaudy jewelry, or potentially controversial things like noserings or unconventional piercings. Don't show up smelling like cigarette smoke, or chewing gum.

9. Do think positively about yourself and your candidacy.
10. Remember to catch your breath and smile.

INTERVIEW FOLLOW-UPS

Another of the more critical components of your interview is the follow-up. This is your opportunity to remind the interviewer of your conversation, and, hopefully, to reinforce your interviewer's impression so that it will carry over to the admissions committee meeting when your candidacy is discussed. Many applicants will overlook or forget this strategic display of manners.

You should not.

In general, you should address a letter of thanks to the admissions director and specific, less formal handwritten notes to some or all of your interviewers. They do get a lot of these notes, so be concise and polite but try to reference the most memorable aspect of the conversation to jog their memory about you. Express enthusiasm for the program one more time, and close. You want to stand out from the masses, and every little well-executed gesture like this can help you to distinguish yourself.

CHAPTER 9

Handling Acceptance, Rejection, and Everything in Between

It's in your moments of decision that your destiny is shaped.
—ANTHONY ROBBINS

WITH YOUR PRIMARY and secondary applications filed and your interviews completed, the waiting game begins again. The wait will seem interminable. Eventually, though, the answers will start to come. This chapter addresses the joy of acceptance, the agony of rejection, and dealing with both to forge a plan that works for you.

HOW TO MANAGE OFFERS OF ACCEPTANCE

Your first acceptance will, no doubt, provide you with one of the peak moments of your life to date. As you read those happy words, a realization will slowly come over you. You are *going* to medical school, and you are *going* to be a doctor.

Congratulations!

If this acceptance is from your top-choice school, or if it is the only acceptance you get, your decision will be an easy one. Say yes and be done with it.

On the other hand, you may be forced to weigh the relative merits of competing offers, none of which are from your top-choice school. This scenario can seriously muddy the waters and provoke significant anxiety.

Let's explore the implications of the various possible acceptance scenarios.

Single or top-choice acceptance

If you got only a single acceptance, or better still, if you got into your top-choice school, your task is easy. Immediately contact the school and accept.

The school will typically follow up their letter of acceptance with a packet that includes an acceptance form and a request for a deposit. Note well, the school must actually *receive* this letter of intent and your deposit check in order to hold your spot. Don't forget to send it in! Make sure it is mailed in a timely and verifiable fashion, and follow up with a call to the school admissions office to confirm that they received it. Once you get that confirmation, you can uncork the bubbly and start celebrating.

As a courtesy to other applicants, if you get into your top-choice school and are certain of your decision to matriculate there, you should immediately contact all other schools that have accepted you or where you still have pending applications and alert them that you have accepted another offer. Do not let your application to other schools hang out there once you have signed a letter of intent just to "see how you would have done" at the other schools on your list. Remember, other applicants are waiting for those spots.

Offers out of synch

There's nothing more exciting than an acceptance. But what if you find yourself looking at an acceptance from a school that isn't your top choice?

Unfortunately, med schools manage their admissions processes differently. Some schools conduct rolling admissions, in which they offer positions to a given number of candidates as they interview throughout the year. Others wait to complete the entire interview season before making any offers. So what happens when a med school using a rolling-admissions process offers you a seat while you have yet to hear from one or more of your top-choice schools that make only end-of-season offers?

First of all, you should *never* turn down an offer of admission without an assurance that you have an acceptance elsewhere. Although the school offering you admission may not represent your top-choice school, you should closely reexamine why you have misgivings about it. Recall what drove your initial ranking of this school, and remember that almost all medical schools provide a first-class education. If you followed our advice, you didn't apply to any schools you wouldn't attend if accepted, so it is worth giving any school that accepts you serious consideration.

Respond immediately to any offer of acceptance in order to maintain an open line of communication. You may politely defer your decision by saying, in writing, "I am honored by your offer of admission, and am carefully weighing my options." The school will then more than likely give you a drop-dead date by which you must give them a definitive answer. Stall as best you can, and use the intervening time to contact the remaining schools ranked higher on your list, alert them of your situation, and ask them to make a decision on your candidacy.

It is perfectly acceptable to contact any schools that you are still waiting to hear from and alert them that you have an offer in hand. This puts some pressure on their admissions committees to review your application and consider accelerating your interview date or to offer you a decision. Your letter should be polite and direct. You should note that you have an offer in hand, and list the reasons you are particularly excited by their school and feel your educational goals would be best met there. At the same time, you should enumerate the unique qualities you would bring to their first-year class.

As you begin to near the drop-dead date on your acceptance offer from the first school, you may even elect to contact some of your most desirable schools directly by phone. Check first to make sure the school does not have a no-call policy. In the absence of such a policy, call and ask to speak with the director of admissions. Relate your quandary and ask for their advice on how to proceed. Again, you are applying subtle but direct and polite pressure to force their hand. It doesn't always work, but it works often enough to make the attempt worthwhile.

If, in the end, you are unable to shake loose any additional offers, get excited about the offer you *do* have. Hopefully your previous research about this school has yielded a growing excitement and eagerness to attend. Remember your broader goals, accept your offer, and know that many opportunities in the world of medicine await you.

Multiple offers

For a lucky few, multiple offers of admission may come streaming in. This is an honor to be handled with humility and integrity.

If you've been accepted at multiple schools, and are confident that you will be declining one or more of those offers, *do so promptly.* Think of it this way: if you're on the wait list at your top-choice school, you're hoping someone else is going to decline their offer in order to give you a chance. You're that someone at somebody else's top-choice school. Have the courtesy to free up the seat so that someone else can share in the joy of acceptance.

Next, consider the merits of your remaining choices. Review your research notes from when you were selecting schools and recall the attributes that attracted you to the different schools. Make a list of pros and cons, then try to determine which program excites you the most. Consider revisiting the campuses of your top two or three choices in order to get a better sense of what life will be like there as a student.

WHAT TO DO IF YOU ARE WAIT-LISTED

In many ways, being wait-listed can be more painful than getting an outright rejection. The med-school application process is so fraught with anxiety to begin with that living in limbo even a little longer seems almost insufferable. On the other hand, many students do, in fact, get accepted off the wait list at nearly every medical school in the country, so there *is* reason for hope. Being wait-listed means you are a competitive candidate, and this gives you an opportunity to state your case more emphatically and demonstrate why your application should be the first one moved off the wait list when the opportunity arises.

Do not react to this situation passively. Spring into action!

First, review your application and the school's attributes. Try to make a compelling case for why you're a particularly good match, and make a list of the unique talents and attributes you offer. State your case in a well-crafted, friendly, one-page letter to the admissions director. Follow up your letter with a phone call and ask if there's any additional information you can provide. Consider asking references or other potentially influential people to make a polite call on your behalf. Some schools have a strict no-call policy, so check first.

Finally, use good judgment here. You're trying to convey your enduring interest to the school. Don't tell them you will accept an offer on the spot unless you are prepared to do so, and don't make a pest of yourself. The line between reiterating interest and becoming annoying is a narrow one. Execute this play well.

In the meantime, you need to make plans to continue with your life. You should assume you ultimately will be rejected, and formulate a plan for the coming fall. Are you going to reapply? Are you going to continue in school? Are you going to look for work? Are you going to travel? Look for pursuits that are engaging, exciting, and continue to build your portfolio of experiences. As you make your plans, be sure to allow enough flexibility so that if you're accepted, even at the eleventh hour in late August, you can matriculate on a moment's notice. There are numerous stories of people being called as late as the second week of classes to come start the year. Don't limit your options such that you would be unable to take such an offer should the chance arise.

COPING WITH REJECTION

Rejection isn't easy to handle, particularly after you've invested years of work in the process. Remember, though, that one of every two med-school applicants fails on his or her first attempt—so you have *lots* of company. It's okay to feel angry and frustrated with the process. Talk it out with your premed advisor, your friends, and your family, and take some time to work through the emotions. Then it's time to pick yourself up and move on.

The first important realization to make is that you are more than just a premed student. You've invested a lot into preparing for medical school admissions, but along the way you've gotten a solid education in the sciences, excelled as a student, and volunteered in your community. These are all things to be tremendously proud of, and these things can form a solid foundation for any number of endeavors, including medicine.

The question that will inevitably haunt you, though, is "Should I reapply?" And you won't be alone.

The answer is simple. If you are truly committed to going to med school, you won't be willing to take no for an answer.

As much as one-third of the med-school applicant pool in any given year is made up of people reapplying. Those students who are accepted the second time around, though, are the ones who put pride aside, carefully scrutinized their application, and sought advice on how to improve their chances.

How do you do this?

Contact each of the schools that rejected you and politely request a meeting or phone interview to discuss what you could do to improve your candidacy. Most schools are very familiar with these requests and are happy to help you identify the gaps in your record and craft a stronger application. Take these suggestions to heart and then make a plan on how to rectify these problems. If your Orgo grade was weak, take it again. If you lacked volunteer or clinical experience, jump in and start shadowing your doctor. Consider pouring your efforts into a master's program that will simultaneously strengthen your application while creating additional credentials if med school ultimately doesn't pan out.

"Make sure you rewrite your essay," Adam adds. "Every school will keep a record of your old application, and it is looked upon poorly not to have changed it year to year. If it didn't work the first time, figure out what is broken and fix it."

Make it clear to all schools in the cover letter of your secondary applications that you are reapplying, and list the specific things you've done to strengthen your candidacy. The key to success on the second go-round is maintaining your enthusiasm and dedicating yourself to becoming a stronger candidate.

"The time between my first and second [applications] helped me grow personally," Deb explains. "During my first round of applications I looked great on paper but was not mature enough to take on the stress of med school. I was nervous and scared interviewing. When I reapplied seven years later, I was much more relaxed and confident. I don't think I looked more impressive on paper, but I had more confidence, which definitely showed in my interview. I knew I was prepared to handle the stresses of medical school."

"Many of my classmates were accepted after their second attempt and they are just as strong, if not better, physicians than those who were accepted their first time," Kate notes. "There are many qualified applicants, but there are limited slots."

You may also decide that you don't wish to reapply.

Perhaps you've made several runs at it and have yet to meet with success. Perhaps your interest in medicine has waned, or along the way you've discovered a new and unexpected passion for a related field. Whatever the case, you should feel no shame in declaring that this is no longer the path for you. Have confidence in yourself and pursue your own horizons, wherever they may lead.

PART THREE

The Preclinical Years

CHAPTER 10

The Five Things to Do Before Classes Begin

In fair weather, prepare for foul.
—THOMAS FULLER

So, YOU'VE RUN the gauntlet thus far. You've begun a life in medicine, pulled through the premed classes, and handled your applications and interviews. Now, the promised land looms on the horizon. Are you ready for landfall and the start of the real adventure?

STEP ONE: CELEBRATE AND RELAX

For many, the glory and relief of being accepted to medical school is quickly replaced by a growing sense of "Oh my God, what have I done? Now I have to go to medical school!"

Stave off the anxiety for a little while and take some time to recognize what you have achieved. You have already demonstrated tremendous dedication and drive, and shown the admissions committee that you have what it takes to be a future physician. Trust their judgment, and your own abilities.

The summer before medical school begins will be the last period of real freedom you will have for many years. Let the stress and strain of the premed process fall by the wayside and take some time to enjoy yourself. True, the next several sections of this chapter will give advice on some specific concepts to consider and tasks to accomplish before classes begin. But even as you undertake these, make sure you take the time to relax and to get excited about achieving a major life goal.

"I think it is incredibly important to relax and try to spend as much time as you can with any significant others you hope to keep around you during medical school," Chris notes. "I was engaged at the time and knew my fiancée was going to be disappointed at how little free time we were going to have together for the next several years."

"I went on vacation before medical school," Deb says. "If I had done anything differently I would have gone on a longer vacation! Enjoy all the free time you can before you start, because it really is a time-consuming and life-altering course you're setting out on."

STEP TWO: FAMILIARIZE YOURSELF WITH THE ROAD AHEAD

The first and most logical impulse you'll experience is to try and get a jump on your studies. Everyone knows med school is a daunting undertaking, and somehow you have this feeling that all that premed course work that you mastered during the past few years isn't going to matter much.

Sadly, your instincts are largely correct. Orgo, Calculus, and their equally unpalatable cousins are a distant memory for most by the time classes start. But take heart! While those classes provided the foundation in the basics that is at some level the necessary base for your clinical knowledge, a continuing fluency in those subjects is unnecessary to get a good start in med school. Do not waste your time reviewing old notes, old texts, MCAT prep books, or basic science concepts. You already know what you need to know.

So what should you do, then?

The best thing you can do is to prepare yourself to study. It is often said that studying in medical school is like drinking from a fire hose. It won't be the intricate complexity of the information that gets you—it will be the sheer volume and the relentless flow of information that will keep you gasping for breath in the first few years of your training. And it will quickly become apparent that the students who are best able to rapidly and efficiently organize and assimilate large quantities of information will be the fastest swimmers in the group.

So you don't have a photographic memory? You can't memorize a three-item shopping list for your trip to the grocery store, let alone an entire medical textbook?

Relax. Few people can. But this is where a little bit of prep work and awareness can give you a real head start on day one.

Take some time to reflect on your sixteen years of schooling and consider the ways in which you learned most efficiently and most thoroughly. Think about the tricks and techniques that you used in the past that got you through your tougher academic course work.

What worked best for you?

Group study?

Flash cards?

Drawing diagrams and flowcharts?

Uninterrupted reading?

Creating outlines?

We all learn best in different ways. Think about how *you* learn best, then decide on the study system that you intend to use to organize and process the information once the fire hose gets turned on in a few weeks. Arm yourself with a mental list of study tools to apply to those impenetrable textbooks you'll soon be prying open.

The next preparatory step you can take is to familiarize yourself with the road ahead. Learn what your first semester classes will be and, if you can, what books you'll be using. Go to the campus bookstore and take a few minutes to peruse those texts. If there's an outline or syllabus required for the class, see if you can get a copy of last year's version to get a sense of the nightly reading load. Forget the details for now. What you're looking for is a basic understanding of the road map for the first year.

Once your head is buried in the books, it will be very difficult to maintain the all-important broader perspective. Understanding how the information you are painstakingly memorizing at the moment fits into the broader medical universe will help you reference and index newly acquired substantive knowledge and allow you to recognize the interconnectedness of your classes and your studies.

Whatever you do, *do not begin memorizing information*. It will be tempting to wade in and start learning.

Don't!

You won't yet know what's important or where to begin, so wait for the first few days of class to get that orientation. For now, just breeze through the chapter headings and get a sense of how the medical textbooks are organized and how the information fits together. You may find reading through the course descriptions in chapter 13 helpful at this introductory phase.

Finally, if you know any students in the class ahead of you, buy them a cup of coffee and ask them a few questions. Thoroughly debrief them on all aspects of the first year—the perils, the pitfalls, the high and low points, and the systems and strategies that worked for them. Remember that their studying and coping mechanisms may be vastly different from your own. Just try to get a general sense of where the biggest challenges are and what, by contrast, may be more quickly breezed through to help you manage your time and priorities.

In the end, remember this: you've been selected from an elite set of applicants to study medicine because you've already proven you've got the academic mettle to handle the task. You'll have your share of tough days, but you'll ultimately chart your own course through the material and come out the other side as an educated and experienced clinician.

STEP THREE: GET MENTALLY, EMOTIONALLY, AND PHYSICALLY FIT

So now that we've crossed studying off your summer to-do list, what *can* you do to prepare?

As we noted, the last few weeks or months before school starts are a rare and precious interlude. If you have the opportunity to be creative with the time, do so.

"I drove cross-country from my job in San Francisco to school in Massachusetts via British Columbia, the Cascades, and the northern Rockies, camping and hiking the whole way," Peter recalls. "Rest and relaxation are paramount, yes, but so are adventure and fitness, introspection and contemplation."

However you spend your time, make getting in shape a priority. As you are about to learn, body and mind complement each other. There is ample evidence that physical fitness leads to higher energy levels, greater satisfaction in life, and better stamina—the very things you will need most as classes get started. The rigors of med school make maintaining any sort of fitness regimen tricky at best, so you should at least start off in good shape. Ideally, you will also discover a basic exercise routine that is convenient and flexible enough to be slipped into your schedule as time allows. All mentors reported regular exercise as one of their key stress relievers during school. Remember, you will need several weeks of regular exercise to effectively make this a comfortable component of your routine, so if you're not already doing so, a regular exercise program is something you should start now.

Finally, spend some time this summer taking stock. You're about to go through a major life transformation. Take some time to consider where you are in life, what you've achieved, and what your hopes and goals are in the near and distant future. Consider your relationships with family, friends, and loved ones. Talk to those close to you about what med school may mean for you. Consider sharing parts of this book, especially part seven, with those you count on as your support network. Tie up loose ends where you can, and seek some inner peace. Starting off calm, confident, and centered will be a great asset when things get tough.

STEP FOUR: FIND HOUSING AND SET UP SHOP

As opening day nears, the competition for local housing becomes intense. Doing some field work up front, either in person or on the phone, will help you assess the market and find the right headquarters for your new life.

Where to live

As with all real estate, start with the essentials: location, location, and location. There is usually an area of town near the medical school and/or major teaching hospitals where modest apartments or small houses are available. Check in with other med students and the registrar's office or the dean's office to find out where most med students live. If you have independent transportation, a larger budget, or requirements not met by these places, you may want to consider places farther afield—but beware. Once classes are underway, time is at a huge premium, so wasted time spent in transit can be a source of major frustration. On the other hand, a little distance can also provide a welcome separation between school and the refuge of home.

"Usually the admissions office of your new school will have some sort of housing folder to get you started," Adam notes. "I was very glad to be located within walking distance of the library and the school for my first two years; this greatly aided my ability to have a variety of places to study. Third and fourth year this was not as important."

Once you've identified a target area, consider your budget limitations. The first decision will be renting versus buying. If you're in a financial position to purchase a home or an apartment at the start of medical school, it may be to your long-term advantage to do so. This is particularly true if you can buy a home or apartment and rent out a room or two to other medical students to help cover the mortgage. The added stress of home ownership and the pressure of a hefty mortgage payment each month, however, may make a purchase less appealing. You should also consider that the real estate market four years from now may or may not allow you to easily or profitably liquidate your investment when it comes time to move across the country for residency. Finally, you should never forget that with home ownership comes maintenance—when the pipes freeze in January on the night before your major neuroanatomy exam, there's no landlord to call. It will be *you* on the phone trying to arrange for a plumber to come out, and *you* stuck with figuring out how to pay for it.

The roommate issue

Your next decision will be whether to live alone or find one or more roommates. Think *very* carefully about this one.

While you may secretly long for the good old college days of keg stands and Wednesday night "It's almost the weekend" parties, these activities won't be conducive to your life in med school. Don't sign up for a living arrangement where your roommates are likely to present you with enticing or unwelcome distractions from your studies. On the other hand, the long hours of solitary study can be very isolating, and some people are aided by the ability to discuss and commiserate with roommates going through a similar experience. As such, some students opt for on-campus dormlike living, which often provides less value for your money in terms of square footage and luxury amenities, but makes up for it in convenience and camaraderie.

If you want to find a roommate but don't know anyone in the new class or the area where you'll be living, your med-school dean's office usually maintains a list of people looking for roommates. As with all roommate situations, be sure to confirm compatibility and carefully discuss how much you're willing to spend and what features you're looking for in a place before signing a lease. Remember to include utilities, phone, renter's insurance, and cable TV (if you opt for that tempting distraction) in your calculations.

"I called the student affairs office and the secretary helped me find other incoming students who were looking for roommates," Carrie notes. "The same secretary also had a list of available apartments in the area. I also thought living within walking distance of school was great, especially during the long Vermont winters when it was nice not to have to worry about shoveling out your car to get to class. I also had fellow students as roommates, which I found comforting."

"All I would say on the roommate question is to put yourself in a situation where you are going to be able to sleep or study anytime that you might want," Chris counsels. "If your potential roommates are likely to be a distraction from studying or are likely to keep you awake when you should be sleeping, get your own place. If you think roommates will serve as a support network, then go that route."

Other housing considerations

Once you've identified a location, settled on a budget, and found a roommate (if you wanted one), you're off to the marketplace. Most major cities offer apartment locator services that tend to have fairly comprehensive and up-to-date listings of vacancies. These services can be good sources of reliable information about building quality and landlord responsiveness, but they usually charge a fee for their services. They also tend to focus on larger, multiunit buildings as opposed to houses or duplexes. Most of your mentors relied on the good old-fashioned Sunday want ads.

If you're moving from far away, obtain newspapers for your city either online or via special order at your local bookstores so you can start perusing the market and making initial calls/appointments well before school begins. As you evaluate the ads, consider the features you're looking for in your new home. The fundamental rules here should be safety, convenience, and simplicity. You've already focused on an area near school; now consider how you'll get around—what's parking like if you have a car, what's public transportation like if you'll go by bus or train, or how easy and safe is it to ride a bike or walk. Graduate student areas don't tend to be in the high-rent district; remember that you will be going to and from campus at *all* hours of the day. You should feel safe coming home in the middle of the night.

Once you've selected a place, make sure that any summer sublettors will be out early enough to allow you to move in at least several days prior to the start of classes to allow you enough time to get settled. Use this time to accomplish such mundane but vital tasks as finding a local bank, getting your telephone and Internet access established, registering your car, and laying in supplies.

Many schools will provide you with or require you to buy a computer before classes start. Get your system up and running before classes begin so you don't have to spend precious hours on hold with tech support.

If you've got the time and can allow a week before classes, take the opportunity to get to know the area a bit, especially if you're completely new to the city. Finding a couple of good restaurants, a place to get your morning coffee, a place to get a bite late at night, and a good place to take a run are important things to do before classes begin.

Your school may also assist you with the transition by offering a planned orientation. This is often a week or so of on-campus and off-campus activities like orientation to classes, honor code review, and dinners with upperclassmen. Don't even *think* of blowing off this orientation if one is offered, as it will likely provide you with an invaluable bonding experience with your new classmates and a good preview of your experience to come.

STEP FIVE: LEARN TO KEEP STRESS AT BAY

Stress is a reality of our everyday, hectic lives, and nothing breeds stress more effectively than medical school. But that doesn't mean you must become overwhelmed by it. As you no doubt know already, stress stems from worrying that you're going to fall short, run out of time, or not be able to complete something. Unfortunately, instead of leading to a solution, stress causes you to dwell on the problem, and in turn, this turmoil causes you to waste way too much time being stressed about being stressed.

The trick is learning to manage the stress of medical school and using a little bit of the pressure you feel as a motivator to keep you moving forward every day.

Keep your perspective

All that takes is perspective and a promise. If you keep perspective on the reality behind the pressure and keep your eye on your fundamental goals, much of the perceived stress will disappear. Remember that you are in med school to become an effective physician, not to ace every test. Nearly every practicing doc has a war story or two about an exam he or she got destroyed on in med school. It's practically part of the experience. Try to remember that you want to learn so you can apply the knowledge in your practice, not just to regurgitate information for one exam. What you are undertaking is a lifelong pursuit—the same concepts you struggle with today will likely still be challenging you and shaping you in new and different ways many years from now. You will not succeed at every turn, but through dedication and perseverance you will grow and thrive. Always remember that *medicine is a vocation, not a life*. You will bring more to your profession and your patients by being a whole person with relationships and interests and experiences outside of medicine than by being the world's most complete walking encyclopedia of medical knowledge. Find a creative outlet, volunteer, and try to set at least one important goal for yourself outside of medicine.

"One of the best things I did with my preclinical years is become extremely involved with community volunteer efforts and community groups," Pete notes. "It was a good way to stay sane and not spend all of my time in Anatomy Lab or a dingy library somewhere."

"Okay," you say. "Got it. I can handle that."

But guess what?

Unless you constantly remind yourself about this, you'll be overwhelmed within two weeks of the start of med school. That's where the promise part comes in.

It's great to start off feeling balanced and in control, but the real work, the real test, is keeping that perspective once you're down in the trenches. When you're feeling overwhelmed, it's tempting to ignore this perspective and focus on nothing but med school. When you find yourself slipping into this pattern (and *trust* us, you will!), force yourself to stop.

Just stop everything you're doing and take a time-out.

Drop back and force yourself to remember why you're doing all this. Remind yourself of the roots of your passion. This may mean taking time *away* from the books, instead of strapping yourself permanently into a chair in the library. Figure out what it was that you did that put you into a state of upset, and strive to avoid falling into the same pattern next time. We're not suggesting that you should blow off your work. All we're saying is that you should—in fact, you *must*—strive to find a balance. Be sure to get your exercise, your sleep, and to get off campus on a semiregular basis to recharge.

"I made an effort to go to class every day," Chris says. "I did this more because I knew if I did not drag my butt out of bed I would sleep until noon every day, not because I got a whole lot out of class. After class I would try to get in a few hours of reading but also make an effort to work in some exercise in the afternoon. I would go home and have dinner with my wife every evening, making sure to spend at least an hour with her, and then take off for the library to study until about midnight."

Remember, this is a marathon and not a sprint.

Get organized and stay organized

That brings us to the second important stress management tool: getting organized and staying organized. The absolute *key* to juggling all your academic requirements and still finding time for yourself lies in good organization and planning. This can be a daunting task. That's why it is important to *start* organized. If you start organized, it'll be easier to stay organized.

The most important organizational tool to acquire is a good calendar reference. It doesn't matter if it's a day planner, a PDA, or a sheet of paper on your wall at home—just make sure you have a good daily and monthly calendar that you *constantly* keep up to date. Once you get class schedules and outlines with test dates, make sure all of those critical dates go onto the calendar immediately. As you add group meetings, group project assignments, and other obligations, make sure everything gets captured immediately on this calendar so nothing falls through the cracks. Get in the habit early of relying on this calendar, keeping it current, and consulting it when you get up in the morning and right before you go to bed at night. Doing so will not only remind you of important deadlines and events, it will give you the peace of mind to know that you're not forgetting anything and help you to relax.

Armed with proper perspective and the organizational tools required to maintain your balance, the last piece of the puzzle is to make sure you actually apply these tools. This may mean budgeting in some time for self-evaluation. One of the best resources can be someone close to you—a friend, a family member, a partner—anyone who can watch you day-to-day from an outside perspective and give you feedback on how you're weathering the storm. When they reach out and tell you you're overstressed, working too much, ignoring too many things in your life, your immediate and natural response will be, "Duh, of *course* I'm overstressed . . . I'm in medical school, I've got three tests next week, and I can't learn anatomy." All that may be true, but *listen* to them. Sit down with a calendar and carve out time to keep moving forward with your studies, but don't forget to budget in some much-needed personal time. Carefully consider your current work priorities and expectations and ask yourself if they are truly reasonable.

"Time management is the key!" Kate insists. "Everyone has the same amount of information to learn, but those who can budget their time efficiently are successful and have pleasant memories of medical school. Make sure you have time designated to yourself and your family, and stay well-rounded. This will help you focus on your studies and have a successful career."

Be ready to practice damage control

Last, you should develop a mental checklist that you will call upon to help you when things go awry. When a crisis develops, don't panic. There aren't many mistakes or problems that can't be corrected. First, help yourself; see if you can identify the problem and institute a solution. This will be a move in the right direction so that when you enter the next step, enlisting outside help, you've already shown you're committed to making things right. Help can come in many forms, but remember that no one is more aware of how stressful med school can be than the faculty at your school. Most of your professors have spent years watching class after class struggle with the same elusive concepts, and seen people make every kind of mistake and experience every kind of breakdown there is to experience. Keep that humbling thought in mind. If you feel yourself slipping or are worried about how things are going, be sure to reach out to the available resources at school. Your professors can direct you to additional study resources, recommend alternate texts or methods of study, or even help set up tutoring. In addition, your school will almost certainly have a range of professional counseling resources for students experiencing trouble either academically or emotionally. In short, when you feel you're wandering off course or losing control, swallow your pride and reach out for help. It's closer than you think, and the sooner you seek help the faster you can get back on track.

But, you say, everyone is stressed to the max and feels like they're sinking. How do you really know when you're in trouble? Take a look at the following list of symptoms:

- Flunking first-term tests
- Uncontrollable urge to cheat or cut corners
- Social and emotional isolation or thoughts of suicide
- Substance abuse or other abusive behaviors
- Unexplained absences from required functions
- Reports from peers that something's amiss with you
- Daily visits, for whatever reason, to the Dean of Student's Office

If you're displaying or feeling any of these symptoms, or if you can't shake the nagging sensation that you're sinking faster than you can bail water, it's time to reach out for help.

CHAPTER 11

Funding Your Med-School Education

*Can anybody remember when the times were not hard
and money not scarce?*
—RALPH WALDO EMERSON

SHOW ME THE MONEY!

THE ACTUAL COST of your medical education obviously depends on which school you attend. According to the most recent AAMC figures, the average cost of a public medical-school education is about $27,500 per year, while the average cost of private medical school is nearly $44,000 per year.

The AAMC also reports that the average debt load for a graduating medical student is slightly more than $100,000 at a public school and $130,000 at a private school. That's an overwhelming sum of money to most people. In 2007 those numbers are expected to increase to $120,000 and $160,000, respectively. Still, an investment of time and money in a medical degree remains a sound long-term investment.

Funding your medical education is a complex process that warrants your dedicated attention and study. Once again, the AAMC Web site (www.aamc.org) provides a wealth of resources for explaining and evaluating your options. There are three sources of financial aid for med students—scholarships and grants, loans, and work-study. Scholarships and grants are blocks of money awarded on the basis of need or merit that do not need to be repaid. Loans fall into one of two subcategories: subsidized or unsubsidized. Subsidized loans do not accrue interest while you're in school, while unsubsidized loans begin accruing interest immediately. Finally, work-study jobs pay you an hourly wage and may apply some of that wage toward your tuition bill.

"One thing I wish I had done was to apply for more scholarships—or any scholarships, for that matter," Deb notes. "There were several people in my class who won scholarships during medical school. Scholarships are out there—you just have to look for them."

Typically, a med student's financial-aid package is derived from a mix of these sources. When you begin school, you will likely have a meeting with the institution's financial-aid advisor. He will have you complete the Free Application for Federal Student Aid (FAFSA) form ahead of time to determine your need, your available funds, and your qualifications for different types of aid. This form will look at your prior student loans, your recent tax returns, your parents' tax returns (depending on your age and independence), and any other financial obligations you have. The financial-aid advisor will help you design an optimal package of funding for your complete education.

Take these meetings seriously, ask lots of questions, and take lots of notes. Managing financial-aid packages can be a complicated task, and staying on top of your aid and the requirements of your various funding sources is imperative. Missing deadlines, missing payments, or failing to meet loan criteria can have dire long-term consequences that could affect your future credit rating and purchasing power.

Scholarships and grants

Your first step should be determining if you can get any money for free—that is, scholarships and grants. Your financial-aid advisor will have a list of scholarship and grant money that he is familiar with, but that should not be the end of your search. Scour the Internet for lesser-known scholarships, and check for available resources in your home and med-school communities. Many civic organizations such as Rotary International offer scholarships for students pursuing a medical degree.

"A five-hundred-dollar Grange or Rotary scholarship may not seem like much, but it is that much less that you have to pay off down the line," Pete notes. "When you calculate the accrued interest that the five hundred dollars would have tacked on over time, you'll realize the value of that scholarship. Every little bit helps."

Consult the appendix (page 271) for more resources to pursue in your search for scholarships.

Subsidized and unsubsidized loans

Everyone is eligible for some degree of federal aid. The primary source for this money is from Stafford and Perkins loans. Stafford loans come in the subsidized or unsubsidized flavors as previously described. The Stafford interest rates are set annually and calculated by the Department of Education based on the 91-day Treasury Bill return. The Perkins loans are similar need-based loans but are shared by the federal government and your school. All the loans go into automatic repayment six months after you graduate from medical school. If you are enrolled in a residency program after graduation, you may have the option to defer your loan payments until after completion of your residency. The AAMC Web site offers the most complete breakdown of the various repayment and deferral programs currently available, so check it for the very latest information.

Most private financial aid is offered by major lending institutions and is coordinated through the financial-aid office at your school. As a student, you will also have an on-campus mailbox constantly stuffed full of fliers from these companies. Their rates tend to be higher and come with more fees and penalties. However, private loans often play an important role in making up the difference between your maximum federal aid and the actual tuition cost. More information regarding private lending sources is usually available through your financial-aid office.

Impact of personal or family resources

The degree to which family or personal resources will play a role in your financial-aid package varies from school to school. Now that you're out of college and living on your own, it may seem ridiculous to think med schools would consider your parents as a source of tuition funds (and if *you* find this notion outrageous, wait until you hear what your parents say on the subject!). Nonetheless, for some of you, family resources may be identified as a source of tuition funds, and if you can't obtain these funds from family, you'll have to look to alternative personal loans to meet the funding gap.

Work-study programs

The work-study program is better suited to undergraduate education, where your copious amounts of free time could be applied to campus jobs. The reality in medical school is that your free time is so limited that you just can't take on a regular campus job; *any* outside work requirements are a distraction to be avoided if at all possible. If work-study is your only option, try to find a way to make the experience both a source of tuition money and an opportunity to get involved in research or other activities on campus that can further your education and strengthen your resume. Most med students who do work-study end up working for the note-taking services compiling lecture notes. If you're considering signing up for a work-study project, be realistic about the time requirements. When possible, talk with students who have done the same type of job to assess its feasibility.

LOAN REPAYMENT PROGRAMS

Financial-aid considerations do not end once your grants and loans have been secured. There are also a number of ways to get your loans repaid for you. One of the more common is a commitment to the armed forces. By signing up for a branch of the military for a period of years, you can get the armed services to pick up the tab for medical school. If you're interested in the military, this can be an extremely cost-effective way to go. Be aware, however, that your choice of specialty or the location of your training may, in part, be dictated by what the military needs. Research these programs carefully before you sign up. Another repayment option is the National Health Service Corps. This federal program offers loan repayment to med students in exchange for a period of service in a medically underserved community. For primary-care doctors attracted to rural living, this can be an extremely attractive and cost-effective approach.

BUDGETING

Figuring out how to fund your tuition and expenses is only half the battle. The other half is being conscientious about managing your personal finances while you're in school. After tuition is paid, there's usually only a relatively modest sum left to live on. Through careful budgeting, you can not only keep yourself in check and minimize your debt burden but you can also effectively stretch your dollar. Remember, though, med school is a demanding experience—it's neither healthy nor fun to try to survive on ramen noodles and free saltines from the nurses' station. You have to grant yourself *some* semblance of a regular life.

Be especially careful about your use of credit. The credit card is often the medical student's nemesis. It becomes frighteningly easy to charge your worries away, blithely ignoring the ever-escalating balances. You can't defer these payments, and the rates are *astronomical.* Do not be tempted. If you cannot control your credit card spending, cut your cards up immediately. There's simply no quicker way to get yourself into a deep financial hole. If you're having trouble living within your budget, talk to your financial-aid advisor to get advice.

"My advice is not to spend excessively in school," Pete advises. "Live simply so that after medical school you can simply live."

RECORD KEEPING

Perhaps the most important thing you can do with respect to your financial aid is to keep good records. This is confusing stuff, and the stacks of statements alone can become overwhelming. Develop a clear understanding about all of your funding sources, make files for each one, and keep up-to-date on the terms of the funds, how much money you owe, current rates, current repayment terms, and whom to contact with questions. Ideally you should review your financial-aid package at least annually with your financial-aid advisor. (You will likely have to do this anyway, since you have to complete a new FAFSA each year.) In between these annual checkups, you should consider starting each school vacation by visiting your aid files and making sure your paperwork is current. Good planning in your final year of med school will also ensure an easy transition to internship and beyond.

CHAPTER 12

Getting Off to the Right Start
in the Preclinical Years

The beginnings and endings of all human undertakings are untidy.
—JOHN GALSWORTHY

GETTING OFF ON the right foot on day one is crucial. We've already laid out a series of strategies for setting up your life and getting your feet under you before school begins. We'll now move on to provide a road map of classes and actual, day-to-day survival tips.

As mentioned previously, there are many different flavors of medical-school curricula. The following sections will describe a traditional curricular approach. The systems and problem-based approaches used in some medical schools are variations on this theme, but they ultimately rely on presenting the same knowledge and roughly the same progression of ideas and understanding.

GOAL OF THE PRECLINICAL CURRICULUM

The goal of your preclinical curriculum is to provide you with a logical foundation of medical knowledge. In your first year, you will start with the fundamental structure and function of the body— Anatomy and Physiology. These courses will take you from the functional organelles of individual cells all the way through complex arrangements of tissues and organ systems. In the second year you will begin to study the impact of disease on the body—Pathology and Pathophysiology. You will also begin to develop a framework of Therapeutics. Each of these subjects will be covered in more detail in the next chapter. As dry as some of this can be, mastering this material is fundamental to your success, as it provides you with the knowledge base you will call upon for the rest of your career.

ESTABLISHING A STUDY STRATEGY

It is essential to develop and adhere to an effective study strategy from the outset. As mentioned in chapter 10, taking the time before school starts to think about the way you learn best can provide useful insights into the most effective way to handle the mountain of information that lies ahead of you. That said, there are three basic approaches to learning in medical school, represented by three typical medical students: Larry, Curly, and Moe. Follow the examples below to see these approaches in action.

Larry the Lecture Hound

Larry is a straight arrow who grew up wanting to be a doctor. He got accepted to medical school right out of college and is eager to jump in. He went to every class he took in college and was a teacher's assistant. He was captain of the soccer team and president of his fraternity. He wasn't much of a reader in college but managed to glean everything he needed from lectures, even without taking notes.

Now Larry has leapt into his med-school classes.

"Whoa, these classes are different! The lectures don't quite cover everything, and they move so fast that detailed notes are tough to take."

Plus Larry is in lectures six hours a day. He tries to review his notes before the weekly quiz but they are fragmentary and incomplete, and often he can't see how the minutiae fit into a bigger picture.

Then someone tells him about the note-taking service. Turns out that guy in the back with the video camera isn't some film-school geek shooting a documentary. He's actually a classmate whose work-study job is to videotape all lectures and catalogue them for the lecture service. Furthermore, Larry notices that every day there's a different person sitting next to him with a laptop, typing away. Turns out this person is adding daily notes to the detailed course outlines, which are also catalogued for the lecture service.

Hmmmm!

A lightbulb goes on for our friend Larry. He can sit in class and glean what he can from the lecture. Then he can review the detailed notes from the note-taking service. For any concept that still doesn't make clear sense, he can fast-forward to that portion of the video-tape and review the professor's comments on the subject. Finally, because the lecture notes are integrated into the course outline, he can identify which areas weren't really covered in class and (gulp) hit the books to cover these concepts.

The only problem with Larry's approach is that all of this will take *hours* every day. Larry has just experienced the stark reality that most people go through in their first few months of medical school—this ain't college anymore. The volume of information is *much* larger. Lectures alone won't cover all the material, so you are forced to do a major portion of your studying independently in order to assimilate and understand the information and how it fits together. Not only will you be required to use the information on tests, but you'll quickly realize that you are building a pyramid of knowledge, and unless you put these fundamentals securely into a foundation, the subsequent concepts and information won't make sense.

But Larry's plan to rely on the note service and videotapes is, in fact, an excellent one. It will provide a structured and detailed review of the information, and it is well suited to the learning style that he adopted in college. However, he will also have to develop the discipline and fortitude to actually sit his butt down and review the notes and the videotape every day after classes to keep himself up to speed.

After a few weeks of stumbling around, a lot of coffee, and one embarrassing episode of anxiety-induced diarrhea, Larry evolves his new study strategy into a very efficient learning tool. He's signed on to the note-taking service, and he's now got it down so that he can review a given lecture in about half an hour, make a list of concepts that he'll want to go over again later, and even look over the outline for the next day so he can anticipate what's coming.

"What worked best for me was being able to read before class, find a way to stay awake in class, and then review the same material that evening," Chris explains. "Mostly I just ended up rereading the note set as often as possible."

Curly the Curious

Curly is a bit of a bookworm. He can quote you Tennyson's poem "Odysseus" in its entirety, even, or perhaps *especially*, after a few too many beers on a Saturday night. He was an English major in college, but he also seemed to excel in a smattering of science classes. He traveled after college working and writing his way through Latin America. In Guatemala, he met some folks that were staffing a rural medical clinic and needed an extra hand. He said he'd be able to help for a week—and stayed for three months. He was incredibly compelled by the work and by the satisfaction and gratification of healing. He decided to think about medical school.

Back in the States, he enrolled in his local college to take his premed classes. They were a drudgery, but having read his way through the major works of Western literature in college, he was adept at burying himself in the books. He found that the classes gave him a good overview, but to really master the material he had to go through it on his own, synthesize it into his own summary, and re-gurgitate it to himself. He was often to be found deep in the bowels of the library or curled up at home, head bowed in a book, making notes hour after hour. He excelled in his premed classes. He was al-most embarrassed when he was named Organic Chemistry Student of the Year. Before he knew it he had completed the premed classes, applied, and found himself staring at a letter of acceptance to his top-choice medical school.

As we join Curly, he's up to his eyeballs in the first weeks of med-ical school. He's tried going to lectures, but finds them alternately boring, confusing, and poorly presented. He takes little information home that he can apply.

"Okay," he says. "It's time to head for the stacks."

He finds a quiet, windowless corner of the library and piles the textbooks up around him. He cracks the first one and sets in read-ing. Two hours later he's covered the first twenty pages—one-fourth of the first lecture in the first class.

"Uh-oh," he says.

If he continues at this rate, some librarian will find his dead and decaying bones years hence, still glued to the chair, only partway through the reading for the first semester. It's time for Curly to adopt a study strategy.

Eventually Curly discovers that the university bookstore has a wide range of review books that summarize the salient points of the texts. He finds he can digest these rapidly, then easily turn them into an outline of his own. Admittedly, they miss some of the finer points, but he finds he enjoys going to the textbook to investigate the details or even pulling up a good review article from the *New England Journal of Medicine.* He tries to look ahead on the outline and identify lectures he should probably go to, but after a few weeks and some calibration, he finds he can cover the material and be adequately prepared for the tests and still go to only half the lectures.

"I realized early on that I did not learn well in lecture format," Ben admits. "I had to read things and put them together on my own to really learn them—so I cut down my lecture attendance and spent the time reading in the library. This was somewhat of a gamble because I was unplugged from the specifics being transmitted in class, but I think I learned much better. I think it's important to figure out how you learn best and try to focus on that method. There's just not enough time in the day to do it all."

Moe the Meeting Man

Moe's a great guy. He's fun, friendly, social, and sensitive. He seemed to do a bit of everything in college. He was a serious student who excelled in his premed classes, but he also played Ultimate Frisbee and managed to get out quite a bit. He was a teacher's assistant during his junior and senior years in college, and he also did some tutoring at the campus center. He found he enjoyed the work, and, perhaps more important, every time he endeavored to teach something to someone, he found that he understood it a little bit better himself. He also noticed that during his premed classes, he particularly liked and excelled in the lab sections, in part because he had some excellent lab partners and they all had a blast working through the experiments and writing them up. In fact, to Moe, the labs were the only part of his premed classes that weren't a chore.

Upon arriving at med school, Moe astutely befriends his Anatomy group. He's happy to find they're all engaging, personable folks, and everyone seems to enjoy working together. They're all smart—in fact, one of the disarming things about the first few weeks of classes has been discovering just how alarmingly smart some of these folks are. However, Moe finds he can certainly keep up with the pack, and it's very clear everyone is struggling under the gargantuan load of information. Within the first two weeks Moe and his Anatomy group agree they should set up some regular study sessions to review. At first they just review Anatomy lecture and lab, but they quickly discover they should expand their scope to include their other classes.

Over time, they evolve a fairly organic format for their sessions. The exact format varies with what they're covering, but in general they meet initially and divide up the material to be covered, then arrange their next meeting. They spend the intervening time going to classes and preparing the information they're assigned. At the group meeting they each present their area of review. Some folks make diagrams, some folks develop mnemonics, and some folks make worksheets. As each person presents, he or she gets peppered with questions from the rest of the group. Over the space of several hours they are able to concisely review the entire block of material, and everyone gets handouts and notes to take home to study later.

Then the first Anatomy test hits.

Moe walks in feeling confident, knowing he and his group have reviewed the material in depth and have done a good job with the dissections. He breezes through the first ten questions because they cover a section of the hand that he himself presented to the study group. His clever, albeit lewd, mnemonics quickly leap into his head, and the diagrams he made help him connect all the pieces.

So far, so good.

But when he moves on to the forearm sections, he starts to get stumped. His friend Jane presented the material at study group, and it all seemed clear at the time. But now her diagrams seem fuzzy in his head, and while he can remember the phrase someone used for a mnemonic, he can't remember what it stood for. Is that tag on the *flexor digitorum profundus,* or is that the *flexor carpi radialis*?

Uh-oh.

Wait, that could be a nerve, not a tendon . . .

Oh, man.

Sweat starts to bead up on Moe's forehead. He tries to remember the lecture, but the professor flew through the diagrams from the textbook, so his notes were sketchy at best.

Needless to say, Moe does not do particularly well on the first Anatomy exam. The good news is nobody does. Nobody ever does well on the first Anatomy exam! But he does notice that the Anatomy Lab group next to his seems to excel. This is odd, since they don't talk much and don't seem to work well together. He sees them at all hours distributed in different parts of the library, working individually. Hmmm . . .

Moe reviews his test results and is pretty bummed. He aced parts of it, but in whole stretches he got next to nothing right. He feels there's no way he can survive a semester of this. He and his group studied for *hours* before the test. Everyone had produced such excellent, detailed study guides. If he didn't learn it then, how the heck would he ever learn it?

Drowning his sorrows in a cup of joe and trying to summon enthusiasm for the coming day's onslaught of lectures, Moe runs into an upper-level student he knows. She asks him how it's going so far.

"Great!" he says. "Except . . ." and he fills her in on the first test.

She actually laughs.

"Man, I remember *bombing* that test," she says. "I cried for an entire night. I was sure I was unfit to be a medical student, let alone a doctor. Then someone gave me the one piece of advice that saved me, and continues to save me to this day: don't study the information, *own* it. Study groups are great, but they can be passive. If you work with a study group, you also have to work through the information yourself because your study group ain't gonna be there on the test helping you with the answers."

Moe's friend is right.

Moe had sat through hours of study-group presentations and felt like it all made sense at the time, but he'd only flipped through the lecture outlines and the handouts from the group in preparation for the test. When push came to shove at test time and he was standing in front of the cadaver, he could not reproduce any of the information he had not directly prepared himself. Maybe this group thing wasn't working out so well after all.

For the next test, Moe tried to prepare all on his own. He found at test time he had a much better overall grasp of the material. However, there had been so much to review that despite spending every waking hour with his nose in a book, there was just no way he could master all the information himself.

Over the next few weeks, Moe and his study group evolved their style into an efficient machine. Others in the group had reached the same conclusion: the relatively passive nature of the group-study approach meant that unless you took time to test yourself and master the material presented by others, it was wasted effort. So, in the end, Moe's group scaled back the number of hours they spent in group study, attempted to develop useful, high-level study aids for each other, and spent a lot of time testing and retesting each other. This overall strategy ended up working very well with Anatomy, and it was easily adaptable to other courses as time went on.

Moe still studies with his group, but he has also come to appreciate the hours he spends mastering the material and owning it. He finds if he reviews, memorizes, and tests himself even before the study-group meeting, he takes more away from the study group, and he can better use the group time to rely on his peers to explain the concepts that are toughest to him. Since they all have different areas that challenge them, they manage to efficiently uncover and smooth out the major bumps on the curricular road.

"I got by with a lot of help from my friends," Deb says. "We had a small group, five of us, that got together regularly before tests and studied. Occasionally someone would have flash cards or make up a flow sheet or chart to share with the rest. Mostly we would go over old exams and the questions would spark discussion or point out weak areas we needed help with. Among the five of us, someone would usually know the answer or be able to explain away the confusion."

Obviously, these are just a few whimsical examples of different med-school study strategies and the advantages and potential pitfalls of each. You will no doubt craft your own. The important point here is not what type of studier you are nor what strategy you ultimately adopt. The important point is recognizing that you will be challenged by the material in med school like you've never been challenged before, and it is *crucial* that you think about and develop a working, effective study strategy early on in your first semester of med school.

It should also be noted that none of the strategies outlined above adopted one of the critical long-term survival strategies endorsed by many of your mentors—using the USMLE board review books as you go along. You will be required to pass the USMLE Step 1 and 2 Exams while in medical school. These will be major rites of passage, so you may as well prepare for them as you go.

Get a good Step 1 book in the first few weeks of classes and make a habit of digesting the relevant material and testing yourself on it as you go along. Make some flash cards that you can use to review both for your class exams and for the USMLE.

All of us wish that we had done this earlier. Learn from our mistakes. Start now.

DECIDE ON A SCHEDULE AND STICK TO IT!

Your study schedule will be almost as individual as your study strategy. You will likely have classes from about 8:00 A.M. to 2:00 P.M., so you'll have to fit the rest of your studying and the rest of your life around these hours. Plan on a minimum of three to four hours of independent study a day. Figure out a way to include some time for yourself, preferably by doing something athletic like going to the gym. Determine just how much sleep you can survive on and still remain healthy and productive. Finally, look ahead in your schedule and plan to take blocks of time off—a day away visiting family, or a weekend camping with friends. These will be relatively few and far between, but the anticipation of these breaks will give you hope and something to look forward to during your long hours at the books.

"I am a night person and would routinely stay in the library until it closed," Adam notes. "I would spend Saturday and Sunday mornings doing nonmedical things, and study in the evenings."

"I would often exercise after class, have dinner, and then study for a few hours," Kate remembers. "I tried to leave one weekend night for social events and was committed to studying the rest of the time. I also made sure I got plenty of sleep."

A typical schedule for a day could go something like this: you might get up around 6:00 A.M. You'll eat a quick breakfast and catch up on any last-minute reading. Say you leave the house around 7:00 and head to campus, getting there around 7:15 or 7:30. Cup of coffee in hand, you'll spend a few minutes catching up with friends or reviewing the upcoming lectures before they start. Classes will probably run from 8:00 to noon; several days a week, you'll have labs from 1:00 to 3:00 or 1:00 to 5:00. You'll usually grab a quick lunch while doing some reading, then head home after classes to spend a few hours with your family or friends. Many students try to do as much studying as possible during regular daylight hours and thereby maximize their at-home free time. Sometimes this works, sometimes it doesn't. Many times you'll get a number of good productive hours in, either very early in the morning or in the afternoons, and then do nothing at night. Other times you might start studying at around 7:00 P.M. and work until 11:00 or 12:00. If you're a group studier, your evening sessions will frequently take place back on campus. You may work for a few hours preparing outlines and questions, then get together as a group and go over material for a few hours. Finally you'll hit the sack, and get up next morning to start all over again.

That arrangement would cover most of the week. On the weekends, you'll probably try to take a full day off, but usually this will amount to about a half day off on Saturday and a portion of Sunday. By Sunday afternoon, stress will usually get the better of you and you'll find yourself back on campus getting ready for the week ahead.

Over time, your body will adapt and you'll find you can function pretty well on four to five hours of sleep a night, providing you have the opportunity to catch up every ten days or so. This fact will allow you to adapt to crunch times like exams when you will stay on campus studying until 2:00 or 3:00 A.M., and then be back in class at 8:00. All-nighters work for some, but you're often too wiped out the next day to focus and actually learn. Caffeine will become a mainstay for most. Exercise may be frustratingly sporadic, but at least try to get outside as much as you can, and remember, the more exercise you get, the more revitalized you will be. Some of the most successful students were the ones who are able to adhere to a regular fitness regimen. You simply cannot underestimate the impact regular exercise will have on your well-being and performance during these incredibly stressful times.

"I think the biggest challenge is to keep from feeling overwhelmed," Chris says. "All I can say is, don't try to look too far ahead. Just keep focused on what is in front of you and the rest will take care of itself."

A STUDY TECHNIQUE TOOLBOX

Here's a quick list of tools the mentors used to build their knowledge base in medical school. You may want to consider adopting them as well.

- Flash cards
- Mnemonics (the raunchier the better!)
- Diagrams and drawings
- Old tests for sample questions
- Revising and rewriting your notes
- Commercial course outlines and reviews
- Listening to taped lectures and reviewing prepared note-service notes

CHAPTER 13

The First Year: Normal Systems

Our own physical body possesses a wisdom
which we who inhabit the body lack.
—HENRY MILLER

T HE FIRST-YEAR CURRICULUM is all about understanding how the human body is *supposed* to work. Much of this material will seem a long way from any clinical application, but it will provide a critical context for the classes to come. Your core anatomy training will include Embryology, Human Gross Anatomy, Cellular Biology, and Histology. Mastering these classes will require that you learn a completely new language of anatomical terminology while at the same time developing a multidimensional sense of spatial and structural relationships of the different pieces and parts. Not an easy undertaking, but it's fascinating stuff. Your Anatomy course will doubtless be an experience you will recall for the rest of your life. The rigors of managing such a staggering volume of information, the challenges of surviving new classes with new classmates, and the emotional impact of dissecting a human being will inevitably leave an indelible mark.

Your core physiology training will focus on developing an understanding of the function of individual organ systems and the overall symbiotic function of the body. Course work here will likely include Human Physiology, Biochemistry, Genetics, and Nutrition. It is, for obvious reasons, vitally important that you understand completely the normal function of the human body before you can begin to address the impact and management of disease—and that's the rationale for the organization of the traditional curriculum. Your course work here will build on your growing understanding of anatomy and yield functional insights. The human body is an intensely dynamic machine, and an appreciation of physiology in action is truly awe-inspiring.

THE FIRST-YEAR COURSE WORK

Anatomy

The human body has thousands of named structures. By the end of your first year of med school, you will be required to identify, relate, and understand a good portion of these structures, which are distributed across the eight major systems of the body. Unless you were a taxonomist in college, this information will likely all be relatively new for you. In fact, even if you took an Anatomy and a Physiology class in college, you will be surprised how differently you will study it in med school.

One of the first and most crucial differences will be the presence of a human cadaver. You and your dissection group of four to eight students will examine this body from stem to stern over the course of your Anatomy class. Many people are nervous about this experience, which is understandable. Day one will be difficult, full of surprises and new experiences.

Most med students have never scrutinized a dead, naked body up close.

Whatever the lecturer says to you during the first twenty minutes will be a blur as you stare down in front of you and think, "Oh my God, it's a dead person."

Your first day of Anatomy Lab will be your first truly quintessential medical-school experience, and one that you will remember for the rest of your life.

After the first twenty minutes of adjustment, though, you must face the task at hand. At first, the scalpel will seem awkward in your hand, and the skin will have the heavy, leathery feel of preserved flesh. But after a few hours you will get the feel of the tools, and the diagrams in your dissection manual will begin to come alive. Tissue planes will make sense as you gently pull away layer upon layer of structures, identifying and labeling vessels, nerves, tendons, and the like. At the end of the first session, you will emerge from the lab with the smell of formaldehyde in your nose, with your head spinning, and with no idea how you will possibly be able to get through an entire body at the painstaking pace you took today. The short list of structures you and your group identified on this day will seem confusing and poorly connected.

Take a deep breath. With time, you will begin to formulate a framework for all this information.

Pay attention, during the first few days, to the general introduction to anatomy. Develop a clear sense in your head of the organizing hierarchy. Use a chalkboard, a white board, or a blank sheet of paper and make sure you can reliably diagram the eight anatomic systems and some of the basics under each one. This diagram represents the systems-based view and will be a fundamental organizing principle for every single anatomic fact you learn.

As you begin to delve into the details of each system, however, you will rapidly arrive at the conclusion that there are at least two other perspectives beyond the systems view that will be fundamental to your mastery of anatomy.

The first is the *structural* perspective.

You must spend time understanding and memorizing the new vocabulary of structural relationships. You must learn to describe the location and orientation of any given structure. It's great to know that the bladder is part of the urogenital system, but it's even more important to understand that it is a pelvic organ and not a peritoneal organ, that it sits directly posterior to the pubic symphysis, that it is surrounded by the vesical fascia, and that it is supported inferiorly by the pubovesical ligament and pelvic fascia. You must know where the ureters that carry urine from the kidneys enter the bladder. Most important of all, you must develop a three-dimensional memory of the bladder and all its parts and connections so that, as you learn more and more facts about this system and its many subcomponents, you can visualize and understand the structural interrelationships. This is not an easy thing to do. You must take time to study diagrams, dissect the parts from your cadaver, and prove to yourself that you can essentially recreate the anatomy for yourself.

Finally, you must learn to put system and structure together to develop a *functional* perspective of anatomy.

In order to reach out your hand and bring the day's eighth cup of coffee to your tired lips, your central nervous system must recognize the image of coffee in your brain, recognize emotions of longing, and send signals down your motor cortex, through your spinal cord, and out via your brachial plexus nerves to the flexors and extensors of your arm, forearm, and hand. The nerve impulses will trigger a muscular contraction that will shorten the muscles and in turn put tension on tendons, which will then pull on bones. The bones will articulate on joints held together by ligaments. As your muscles fire and your arm moves, your nervous system will come back into action, visually observing the progress and calibrating the nervous impulses until, hallelujah, your hand contacts the warm cup, the cutaneous nerves in your fingertips register a firm warm shape, you grasp the cup, bring it to your lips, and take a long, sustaining drink.

Pretty cool, huh?

The problem is, your body does about a billion different things, and each is a delicate and well-orchestrated ballet of multiple systems and their interacting structural components. It is as complex as it is awesome, and you'll need to know it all.

The trick, of course, is figuring out how to piece all of this knowledge together and develop an efficient way to process, catalogue, and master this immense amount of information.

First, don't panic.

Although it will feel like you could never possibly master even a third of the material you're expected to know, you will—just as legions of medical students before you have done. Surround yourself with the course outline, a couple of anatomy textbooks, and a stack of blank paper. Reflect on the first week's worth of material in the course outline and get a sense of what systems and structures you'll be expected to know. The outline is more than likely organized around the systems model. Understand the system and how its major components relate. Make a checklist of the specific anatomic structures you are expected to know.

Once you've done that, hit the anatomy texts. Most people use Frank Netter's exceptional atlases. You may also find alternate texts such as *Grant's Anatomy* or *Gray's Anatomy of the Human Body* useful to provide a couple of different pictures and views of the same structures. As you study the texts, don't get overwhelmed by the extraneous structures you're not expected to know. In fact, many folks highlight the required structures in their textbooks so they can focus exclusively on them. Closely examine the drawings and describe to yourself in proper anatomical terms the location and structural relationships of the item in question.

Memorize, memorize, memorize.

Make drawings and label them. Copy pictures from the text, white out the labels, and then rewrite the labels from memory. Make flash cards. Quiz yourself constantly. Work with your study group to come up with memorable and creative ways to remember the facts.

Live, eat, and breathe anatomy. It is, after all, the cornerstone of medicine.

If you master the systems and structural perspectives, you will surely do well in your Anatomy course. While functional view is also a critical component to your understanding of anatomy, the majority of it will actually come from some of your other course work—primarily Physiology, as well as Cellular Biology and Biochemistry. If you're lucky, your Physiology and Anatomy classes will be integrated and this functional perspective will be presented simultaneously. If not, take those same concepts you've worked with in Anatomy and extend them as you delve into subsequent course work.

"I did not like the members of my Anatomy group very much initially—most of them were very intense," Carrie recalls. "They all thought they wanted to be surgeons and used to fight over who got to dissect. When we were doing the head and neck section, they brought in head lamps, so we could see better. Everyone else in the class thought this was ridiculous and called my group 'team surgery.' I often felt intimidated during class and did not feel it was a good learning environment for me. I tolerated my group, but I did most of my studying/learning after class with a few friends. The funny thing is that none of them went into surgery. And, by the end of med school, I was actually very close friends with some of them."

Physiology

Your Physiology course will provide the critical functional context for the anatomy you've just started mastering. Here, you will study the complex and dynamic interplay among body systems that produces our biologic imperatives as living, growing, learning organisms. Again, the scope is, at first, bewildering. Hold on to your hat and, as always, begin by developing a macroscale blueprint for the information. Most of the anatomic systems you studied will directly translate into physiologic systems. Start with these concepts and extend your understanding to more complex physiology as you uncover functionality that spans multiple systems.

The structural perspective in Physiology goes one level deeper than in Anatomy. Your Gross Anatomy class deals primarily with specific tangible structures and organs. Your study of physiology will extend all the way from an appreciation of cellular biology and biochemical signaling pathways up to integration of entire organ systems. The study skills and multidimensional thinking cultivated in Anatomy will serve you well here. Make sure you understand each level of the tree and can adequately define the cellular and anatomic entities involved as well as their contribution to the overall functional process.

As with Anatomy, it is useful to organize the information along functional, anatomic, and systems perspectives so that you challenge your understanding and integration of the information. Diagram, discuss, rehearse, and test yourself independently and with your group.

Biochemistry

You were hoping that all that premed crap you slogged through would be a distant and disturbing memory, right?

Well . . . not quite.

Your Biochemistry class will reunite some uncomfortable points of Organic Chemistry with those dreaded metabolic reaction chains (the Krebs cycle and the like) from your Intro Bio class. On the one hand, this course can be onerous, since it proves to be yet another memorization marathon. On the other hand, most of your mentors recall this class as being one of the easier ones since they had previously seen much of the same information in their premed classes.

If you take the time to integrate your Biochemistry studies with the structural and functional framework you've developed in Anatomy and Physiology, you will be impressed by the perspective it yields about the molecular underpinnings of who we are and how we work. As you will discover, our most complex thoughts and creative moves are, in fact, simply the end result of some insanely dynamic and well-orchestrated chemical reactions. As we've said before, getting this perspective on the knowledge you are acquiring is *critical* to your success in med school. You need to see and understand how everything fits together into the big picture.

Remember—always—that it is first and foremost about *learning*.

There are numerous approaches to studying biochemistry. Many students opt to list and diagram reactions. Search your med-school library for Jack G. Salway's *Metabolism at a Glance*, an excellent text that beautifully diagrams entire reaction chains. The book takes the cascades of biochemical reactions and graphically orients them to the relevant cells and organelles, giving you a unified functional and anatomic view of the process. By studying these diagrams and re-creating them in your own hand, you should be able to retrieve them reliably when test time comes.

While you will be required to memorize these reaction chains for the tests, and a few of them for the boards, you will never see them again in your training or clinical practice. To this end, the most important concepts to take with you from your study of biochemistry are an appreciation for the fundamental molecular building blocks, an understanding of the different areas of metabolism, and an in-depth knowledge and familiarity with the basic signaling pathways. While you may need the details for the tests, don't worry so much about the details in the long run. Understanding the concepts and broad outlines of pathways in these areas will serve you well as you begin to study Physiology, Pharmacology, Genetics, and Nutrition.

Biochemistry is another great subject to review in the USMLE Step 1 board review books as you go through the class. You may have access to old tests from your classes, but you'll likely discover that many of the things your professor emphasizes may not be empha-sized on the boards and, conversely, that there may be some material on the boards that your professor barely covered in your class. Take the time *now* to make your board-review flash cards, use them for your Biochem tests, then tuck them away until your second year when you can use them again to review for the Step 1 boards. Killing two birds with one stone in this fashion will make you a very, very happy med student down the line.

Trust us.

Cellular Biology

Cellular Biology is essentially Anatomy and Physiology at the mi-croscopic level. Here, you will begin to appreciate how and why tis-sues function harmoniously as organs and organ systems. You will come to understand the life cycles of different cells of the body, how we age, and how we renew ourselves when problems arise. You will investigate the body's immune system and how we wage war on invaders—and sometimes on ourselves. You will see cancer in action and examine why it's so hard to treat.

Much of cellular biology hinges on how cells react to their local environment and communicate with each other. To this end, your studies should focus on these interactions and signaling pathways. There are numerous computer animations available online and at your medical school to help illustrate these concepts. It is worth your while to seek out, find, and use these animations. In many cases a single brief animation will literally be worth thousands of words in the textbook in terms of its value to your understanding of the concept.

Like biochemistry, cellular biology is an area only lightly tested on the USMLE Step 1 Exam, so you should use your board review book contemporaneously with your course text and make sure you hit all the high points. Make your flash cards now, use them to prep for your classroom exams, and then put them away so you won't have to reinvent the wheel come boards time.

Neurobiology

The brain and the nervous system are among the toughest challenges of first-year med school. Remember when we said that most of the challenge of med school was in volume, not complexity? Well, here you get volume *and* complexity.

The course typically starts with the brain and its many subcomponents. You will learn the basic architecture, the functional units, and how they relate. You will probably also review the embryologic development of the nervous system again. Once you have a sense of which area does what and how they communicate, you will begin to investigate the major input and output tracts. How do the twelve cranial nerves control things like eyesight, hearing, taste, and smell? If you step on a nail, how does the sensory input in the skin on the sole of your foot travel from the cutaneous nerves to the large peripheral nerves to the ascending sensory tracts of the spinal cord and into the brain? In turn, how does this sensory stimulus generate both a feeling and location of pain in the brain as well as an immediate reflex that requires no thought control?

Not only is Neurobio one of the most fascinating classes you'll ever take, it's also a crucial one. As such, be certain to take the time to get the anatomy memorized, then start to overlay your functional understanding on that. Draw diagram after diagram. Test yourself repeatedly. Test your friends. Make your friends test you. The only way to get good at these concepts is to test your understanding of them.

You may never forget the weekly tests from your Neuroanatomy class that will have you tearing your hair out over the fine distinctions contained in A-through-K multiple-choice questions. Learned properly, however, the course material will provide you with an appreciation for and a fundamental understanding of the nervous system that will, on many occasions, guide your clinical practice.

Embryology

Embryology is, unfortunately, a class often given short shrift by medical students. Since you've already poured your heart and soul into mastering Anatomy and Physiology, mustering the strength to comprehend and memorize the embryologic evolution of each body tissue can feel like cruel and unusual punishment. Nonetheless, an appreciation for this critical process will enhance your understanding of disease later and give you further respect for how the human body functions.

Start with the basic unicellular embryo and begin tracing each dermal layer's development from there. Focus on how each layer of the evolving embryo differentiates into specific organ systems. There are some pretty good animated models available online and at most medical schools that can provide a more visual guide to the migration of cells and tissues. This is definitely a subject area where looking into a USMLE Step 1 board review book will ensure that you retain the critical information you will need later on the board tests. With the exception of genetics and some specific clinical specialties, though, you will probably seldom use your knowledge of embryology in day-to-day practice.

Genetics

You don't have to be more than a casual observer of the popular media to realize that genetics is a hot topic both in medicine and in society more generally. Seemingly limitless in potential yet fraught with ethical controversy, this relatively new field continues to expand like a supernova. As we learn more and more about the human genome, we begin to see that almost every aspect of our anatomy, physiology, and pathophysiology is tied to our genes.

Hope truly lies buried in that code.

Your medical-school class on genetics will likely be somewhat more rudimentary. Most curricula are struggling to modernize and stay abreast of the staggeringly rapid developments in the field. Strive for an understanding of the fundamentals of Mendelian and non-Mendelian inheritance, as well as the basic techniques used to determine and decipher a genetic sequence. You will take an in-depth look at cell division and genetic inheritance, which was first covered in your college Biology course. You will also begin to look at common dysmorphisms and understand their genetic basis. Again, it is important to review the relevant USMLE Step 1 material and make your flash cards so you don't need to re-create these materials next year.

Nutrition

Yes, this course is more than just the same old food pyramid from your sixth-grade lunchroom wall. In fact, this class will provide you with a wealth of information on the fundamental energy and functional building blocks for healthy metabolism. The class will not only cover the basic dietary components but also make forays into metabolic deficiencies, homeopathic and alternative remedies, and clinical nutritional decision making. This class usually has a relatively light workload and is covered minimally on board tests. Use your board review book to identify and master the fundamentals.

Ethics

Many people consider their Ethics class to be an unnecessary distraction from classes like Anatomy. The truth is, the first-year Ethics course does two things for you. First, it offers you the chance to exercise the half of your brain that has been idling while the scientific/logical/memorize-the-entire-book side of your brain is beaten into submission. Not only does left-brain thinking play an important role in medicine, ethical issues are playing an increasingly significant role in the lives of today's doctors.

No matter what field you go into, as a physician you will often be forced to make choices between what is best for the patient, best for the hospital, and best for your practice. Hopefully your Ethics class will give you some tools to approaching these difficult issues.

Most Ethics classes begin with a fairly dry litany of ethics principles before delving into their application with case-scenarios. With luck, you will have an engaging, small group that can bat these cases around. You will be surprised at how complex some of the seemingly straightforward cases can become and by how different your opinion of the right course may be from that of some of your colleagues. These real-life cases are guaranteed to stimulate good discussion. What you will find especially gratifying, however, is recognizing these same situations and scenarios in your clinical rotations and clinical practice and reflecting on how important many of these lessons truly are.

Introduction to Clinical Medicine—your first patients

Most med schools start you out in the first year with some form of "Introduction to Clinical Medicine." This course is typically a combination of a regular didactic component coupled with weekly clinical exposure. The didactic component of this class will focus on teaching you the fundamental skills of taking patient histories and performing physical exams. While it may seem pretty straightforward, the truth is, it's a very complex skill set that takes years to perfect.

In addition to the basics of what's in a good history and how you should listen to the heart and lungs, the class will also cover the importance of good communication styles, how to make patients feel like they've been heard, how to deal with difficult patients, and how to address communication barriers like language, culture, and disabilities. Many schools will test you on these skills through the use of Objective Structured Clinical Exams (OSCEs). On these tests, you will be expected to interview and examine a simulated patient (actually an actor). Your encounter will be captured on videotape, and you will be scored on the accuracy of the information you collected as well as the style with which you conducted yourself. You will review the tape with a mentor to discuss ways to improve.

In the last few years, the OSCE has taken on a whole new level of importance. Starting in 2002, the USMLE Step 2 Exam began featuring an OSCE component. It is worth your while to pay attention to your OSCE training and develop your skills early in this area. If you practice and approach the simulated patient the same as you would an actual patient, you will do just fine.

For your weekly clinical exposure, you will be assigned to a primary-care provider in the community, and you will spend one afternoon a week shadowing that person in his office or hospital practice. For most students, this is the most riveting, engaging, and gratifying part of their entire first year. In these precious few hours each week, you get to leave the books and tests and facts and figures behind and don the white coat.

Yes, you will fumble and feel awkward and out of place.

Yes, you will embarrass yourself.

But at some point during this experience, a patient will turn to you and say, "So, Doctor, what do you think I should do?" And in that moment, you will realize the amazing gift you have been given by being accepted to medical school. Suddenly, those hours in the Anatomy Lab will begin to possess a poignant sense of urgency. It doesn't make the studying any less hard, but it does give all that hard work unquestionable relevance.

As a final note, we should mention the myriad additional extracurricular clinical opportunities available to you during your first two years. Most students feel that the few hours of time they get with their clinical preceptor each week are like gold. This needn't be the end of your exposure. Most medical schools staff local free clinics for the homeless and underprivileged. They provide a great opportunity for you to volunteer your time, gain more clinical experience, and continue to build your resume as you look toward residency.

A WELCOME SUMMER OFF

In most programs, the summer between your first and second year of med school will be your last gasp of freedom. After the end of your second year, you will roll directly into third year, since the clinical academic calendar runs from June to June. Thus, the few weeks between your first and second year are the last serious block of time you will have to yourself for a long, long time—and possibly ever. Make good use of these precious weeks.

What that means to us is relax and have some fun.

You've worked your butt off to survive the first year, and you deserve some much-needed R & R. Plan a trip or adventure. You needn't do anything medically related unless you want to. This time will not be closely scrutinized on your residency application, so if serving ice cream and traveling to Ottawa end up as your big achievements during this time, that's okay.

That said, there are a few things you could consider doing that may pay off for you later. First, many people have a lucrative skill set from prior jobs that they may be able to jump back into to make some money over the summer. Avoid burnout at all cost, though, so *do not* put yourself in a high-pressure job all summer just to make money. On the other hand, a quick infusion of capital can make living expenses during the second year a bit easier to handle or may even allow you to reduce your debt load.

If you're interested in doing something medical, consider getting involved in research or a clinical or an academic project. Look for something that seems fun and interesting and may reflect a clinical direction you're curious about pursuing. Maybe there's a great lab project getting under way you want to help out with. Maybe there's a medical relief trip being planned to some remote corner of the world that you can plug into. There's no end to the options if you explore your resources. Talk to your favorite faculty members and peruse your med school's Web site. Cold-call people affiliated with your school who are doing things you're interested in. You'll be surprised at how far the "I'm a first-year medical student" credential will take you. It opens more doors than you would think.

Let us emphasize one more time, though—do *not* do something inherently stress-provoking, sleep-depriving, or emotionally tumultuous. The rigors of your medical education should already provide more than enough stimuli in those arenas. Do something fun and engaging and challenging that broadens your perspective and reminds you why you went to med school. Then tuck that inspiration away in your closet for the long, rainy days in the library when all you want is to stop studying.

"We had a wonderful program at my medical school called the Pathway for the Underserved," Pete recalls. "This included funding for language training and international experiences with a coordinator who possessed the most comprehensive folio of international medical programs, volunteer opportunities, and electives I have ever seen. As a result of this program I spent six weeks in Ecuador the summer after my first year, undergoing intensive language training and working in a clinic."

CHAPTER 14

The Second Year: Disease and Medicine

The good physician treats the disease;
the great physician treats the patient who has the disease.
—Sir William Osler

At the dawn of the second year, you will make the transition from studying normal Anatomy and Physiology to studying disease and its impacts on the body. Your course work now will focus on Pathology (a study of the impact of disease on anatomy), Pathophysiology (the impact of disease on the body's function), and Pharmacology (the basics of how we treat pathology and pathophysiology with medications). You will also take Microbiology, in which you will cover the broad spectrum of bacteria, fungi, viruses, and parasites that can wreak havoc on the human system.

Most important, it is during the second year that you will begin to develop the essential framework of clinical decision making and differential diagnosis.

We are taught medicine in the form of lists and tables from the annals of various specific subjects like Anatomy or Microbiology. Patients, on the other hand, know nothing of the science and give us only constellations of symptoms. The art of medicine is in recognizing the patterns of symptoms, knowing the mechanics and progression of diseases in the body, and correctly identifying your patient's illness. These skills will be emphasized during your clinical rotations in the next two years. But it is during the second year that you will begin to develop your clinical decision-making ability by considering differentials as you learn the basics of disease.

Finally, the spring of second year is when you typically take the first step of the U.S. Medical Licensing Exam (USMLE Step 1). This is a major rite of passage and a major undertaking. Hopefully you've followed our advice and have been slowly accumulating study materials with each class you've taken. This will make your preparation for the test infinitely more efficient and enjoyable. Chapter 15 will deal with preparing for and taking the Step 1 Exam in detail.

"Differential diagnosis is the key to life," Deb advises. "Start thinking about this early in your training! Ask why and how about everything you can. I think medical school trains us well to memorize details for multiple-guess questions or to expand on the minutiae of a single disease process quite well. Patients, however, rarely present us with a single disease. More often, they present us with multiple vague symptoms and we must pick one of the several things that may be the cause.

"For instance, in the anesthesia world, a patient under general anesthesia may be hypotensive, but why? Is it because they are dehydrated from being without food or water for the last twelve to twenty-four hours? Is the patient suddenly losing a lot of blood from the surgical field? Are the medicines we are giving, such as the anesthetic gas, vasodilating the patient? Is the patient having an allergic reaction to the antibiotics he is receiving? There are many different choices for the cause of one symptom, and in order to treat the problem correctly you must know the cause. Turning down an anesthetic gas when you haven't even thought of treating the patient's anaphylaxis won't necessarily help you. The larger your differential, the less likely you are to miss something."

THE SECOND-YEAR COURSE WORK

Microbiology

Infectious disease is at the core of many, if not most, human diseases. Even some cancers are thought to have their origin in earlier viral infections. Understanding the spectrum of agents that can affect and infect the human body is critical. The discipline is inherently broad. We are continually discovering wholly new pathogens and observing old pathogens evolving to take on new characteristics.

Your course work in Microbiology will be divided along taxonomic lines. You will have sections on bacteria, viruses, fungi, parasites, and atypical agents. In each section you will learn the members of the group, their mechanism and manner of infection, their lab identification, and the drugs potentially used to combat them. You will also have a lab section that requires you to grow and evaluate microorganisms, and to develop a familiarity with at least the basic lab techniques like Gram staining and microscopy.

The key to mastering microbiology will be . . . you guessed it . . . memorization. If you understand the organizing framework early and start memorizing aggressively, you will develop a structured perspective on the discipline in addition to the specifics of each organism. An excellent reference book by Mark Gladwin and Bill Trattler called *Clinical Microbiology Made Ridiculously Simple* has been the bible of this course for years. Flash cards are also immensely helpful here.

Don't sweat the lab stuff too much—unless you're going to be an M.D/Ph.D. or otherwise have the opportunity to conduct research, you'll probably never use these skills again. Clinically the important lesson will be knowing which tests to order on a given sample and why. Go over your Step 1 review book to get the proper perspective and to help you handle the challenging microbiology questions on test day.

Pathophysiology

In Pathophysiology, you will examine the impact of disease and dysfunction on human physiology. Your mind should still be fresh with your understanding, gained during your first year, of how the body is *supposed* to work. Now you must examine the impact of infection, metabolism, trauma, environment, failure, and aging on these processes. Why does the impact of diabetes extend well beyond high blood sugars? How does cholesterol play a role in heart disease? Why do alcoholics suffer from liver failure?

Your Pathophysiology course work will probably follow the same general sequence you followed in your Physiology course. Obviously this course forces you to review your normal Physiology as well, so take advantage of the opportunity to fill in any gaps or weaknesses and review concepts for the Step 1 Exam. Make sure you have a clear framework for the broad range of diseases presented here. You will rely and draw on the complete spectrum of information you garner in this course for the rest of your clinical career.

This is a key subject in which to use your Step 1 board review books and develop a set of flash cards or another study method that you can rely on to review for the Step 1 Exam.

Pathology

In Pathology, you will review each organ system you learned in Anatomy and begin to understand how it can be affected by disease and dysfunction. You will be investigating the impact of infections, toxins, genetic diseases, injury, and metabolism on the structure of the organ systems. Your lab work will focus on reviewing histologic slides under the microscope and looking at specimens.

This course will review the major anatomic systems and the disease states that affect them. You will learn the microscopic and macroscopic impact of disease on the various organs and tissues. Your didactic review of the material will be supplemented with lab time spent examining whole organ specimens as well as thin sections under the microscope. If you're lucky, you'll also have the chance to observe an actual autopsy—and probably be surprised by how different the newly dead, unpreserved body looks from the cadaver you became so familiar with during Anatomy.

Pharmacology

This class will be your first major foray into therapeutics— treating disease and healing patients. You will start with an introduction to basic pharmacologic principles on how drugs function and how they are distributed in the body. Then you will step through each major drug class, reviewing the different drugs in that class, their therapeutic goals, mechanisms of action, side effects, and appropriate dosing regimens.

There is a massive amount of memorization here. Flash cards are virtually imperative. You will have to review and rereview, test and retest before all the different drugs become familiar enough for you to be able to apply them. Take the time to do this right the first time, as any lingering uncertainty about what a drug class does will be a serious handicap next year when you hit the wards.

That being said, it is also true that these days there are more drugs than any single person can possibly remember, and there's just too much information on each drug to have it all available for immediate recall. There are, however, several useful pocket, PDA, and computer resources that let you instantly look up drugs in the clinical environment (see appendix, page 271). You will come to rely on these tools once you're on the wards. For now, however, good, old-fashioned memorization will provide the conceptual and factual underpinning you need to be effective in the clinical environment. Not surprisingly, this area is also tested heavily on the board exams, and no outside resources are permitted—so you simply have to master as much of this material as you possibly can.

Enjoy your drink from the fire hose.

Human Behavior/Psychiatry

This is primarily a clinical rotation in your third year, and many schools now include a didactic curriculum in basic human behavior during the second year as well. This course is concerned with defining what is generally considered normal behavior and the principles that govern it. You will also spend a significant portion of your time learning how to take a detailed family and social history, and how to develop a basic psychosocial profile of any given patient.

There are really no tricks to mastering this class. The workload is typically low, and the performance is primarily clinical. Enjoy a non-memorization class and an opportunity to explore some of the left-brain concepts in medicine. A healthy appreciation for what drives us as humans and how we react to events in our lives will be an important weapon in your clinical arsenal.

CHAPTER 15

Bringing It All Together:
The USMLE Step 1 Exam

By failing to prepare, you are preparing to fail.
—BENJAMIN FRANKLIN

YOUR PRECLINICAL STUDIES will culminate in the mother of all exams—the USMLE Step 1 Exam. This exam will be unlike any exam you've ever taken before—it is longer, more comprehensive, more detailed, and, frankly, more difficult than anything you have ever seen.

AN OVERVIEW OF THE STEP 1 EXAM

The USMLE Step 1 Exam confronts you with approximately 350 multiple-choice questions in seven one-hour test blocks. And the questions aren't unidimensional like "What nerve innervates the heart?" They are primarily clinical vignettes that force you to pick up on anatomic and physiologic clues that subsequently relate to pathophysiology or pharmacology. Thus, a typical question would be something like this:

"The patient has had two heart attacks and is on a cardiac medication regimen. She presents with right upper quadrant abdominal pain and jaundice. The drug most likely causing her jaundice is . . ."

Your response would require you to know that since she has known heart disease, she's probably on a standard regimen, which would include a cholesterol-lowering agent. From this assumption, you would recognize that among the common drugs in this class (known as the statins) are a group of drugs that lower cholesterol by inhibiting the synthesis of cholesterol precursors. They also tend to cause liver dysfunction and muscle pain as common side effects. In fact, these are some of the most common reasons for patients' intolerance to this class of drugs.

PREPARING FOR THE STEP 1 EXAM

The USMLE truly does require you to bring it all together—that is, synthesize all the information from your preclinical studies into a one-day checkpoint. That being the case, you're probably wondering how you should approach studying for an exam of this breadth and scope.

The old adage is "Two months for Step 1, two weeks for Step 2, and a number-two pencil for Step 3."

This may not quite hold true, but in general it is true that Step 1 is far and away the hardest, Step 2 builds on more clinical data and is easier to approach, and by the time you take Step 3 you'll have enough experience under your belt that you'll find the exam to be fairly straightforward.

If you've followed the advice in this book you should already have a *huge* head start on most of your colleagues. By the spring of your second year, your classmates will be frantically buying board review books, streaming through the pages, and crying in desperation as they realize that (1) half the stuff they studied and memorized for their class work over the last two years is not on the Step 1 test, and (2) the other half that *is* relevant could have been prepared for contemporaneously with their classroom study of the individual subjects—which would have saved them an incredible amount of time and effort.

Now aren't you glad you bought this book?

As you stride into the library, past carrel after carrel of red-eyed, stressed-out students, you'll be confident that that large bundle of your previously prepared flash cards and the well-annotated board review book you've been working with during the past two years as you covered each subject will have you doing just what you should be doing—*reviewing* for the boards, not *learning* for the boards.

An organized and dedicated study plan, however, is still in order. Most med schools offer some protected time to allow second-year students to focus on studying for the boards. If yours doesn't, make sure you plan out a lighter course load or a period of time off to dedicate yourself solely to studying for Step 1. You need to capitalize on the advance work you have already done and identify your areas of weakness.

Listen up, though—and heed this advice.

Take all your class notes, bundle them up, and put them on a high shelf in the corner. Reviewing entire subjects from your notes and outlines is *not* an efficient study strategy.

Not unlike the MCAT, your goal here is to study to survive and thrive on this particular test, not to remaster the subject matter. Thus your study strategy must focus on how to beat the particulars of the test.

You must learn to study smart—not just study hard.

Start with a solid general boards reference book like McGraw-Hill's *First Aid for the USMLE Step 1*. The First Aid series does a nice job of concisely providing the factual information you need to master in order to compete on the boards. The series has been the most popular with medical students for some time, and the authors continue to refine and update the material to stay current with the test.

The book offers little in terms of explanation or context, and its approach is somewhat fragmentary. However, it's an excellent place to start because you can review the material and assess what's familiar and what's not.

Simply put, you need to know *everything* in this book.

At first this will seem like an unreasonable, unwieldy, impossible task. But once you wade into it, you will discover that you already know much more than you thought you did. Go through the flash cards you made in each class and organize them according to the outline of this book. Now review all your flash cards and go through the material in the book at least once. Make a running list of areas in the book not covered by your note cards. This will be your subject-review list for further study.

The next step is to begin testing yourself. Get yourself one of the many board review question banks. You can purchase these either in book form or on CD-ROM. Since you'll be taking the actual test on the computer, we advise you to train with the CD-ROM. Tote around your laptop and work through question sets at your favorite bookstore or coffee shop, at the library, or at home on the couch. Be sure to acquire a test set that has complete explanations of all the answers. Set aside time at the beginning to take at least one complete test block under real-time conditions. Don't cheat and look at answers as you go. This is your self-evaluation.

When you complete and score the test, don't be dismayed by your score—you're only just starting your preparation, and you've got to start somewhere. Now you have a baseline.

Next, go back through the answers to all the questions. Make sure you got the correct answers correct for the right reasons, and make sure you understand the reasons for all the wrong answers. Make note cards to memorize the questions you got wrong. Incorporate these cards into your growing set from the board review book and your previous classes. As you discover subject areas where you exhibit weakness, add them to your subject-review list.

Now take that subject-review list and begin filling in the holes. At this point, if you can't restrain yourself from doing so, you can pull down your course notes and review them. However, a good subject-based board review book will likely do a better job of providing the same context and structure with, again, a specific focus on what's going to be tested on the boards as opposed to what your professor was interested in teaching you.

There are many different series of books available. As mentioned, the First Aid series offers a detailed review of most of the major review books with letter grades reflecting the quality and usefulness according to the editors and prior students, so consult that resource first. Don't get bogged down in reviewing an entire subject unless you really feel you need to. The goal here is to fill in the gaps to round out your complete spectrum of knowledge for the boards. Attempt to be as focused as possible in your subject reviews. Make additional note cards as needed to ensure that you capture and master the material you review.

From this point on, you simply need to keep repeating this same cycle until test day. You should see progressive improvement in your mastery of the material on your note cards, the subject matter in the Step 1 review book, and in your actual sample test scores. You should hit fewer and fewer questions that are stumpers or seem foreign, and you should find your subject-review list shrinking down to none.

"Great," you say, "that sounds like a solid plan. But is it realistic? How much time should I allot for studying?"

This is a fairly individual thing, but as a rule you should allow for at least one full month of solid, 100 percent committed study time.

That means studying every day, for ten to twelve hours a day, for the entire month. That means being dedicated to and focused on the undertaking, and removing as many distractions as possible. This will be a hard and painful push, but it is an important one. The USMLE Step 1 Exam is a critical checkpoint along the road of your medical education, and many of the more competitive residency programs use the score you earn on this exam as an important component of their match decisions. There is no way around it—the only way onward is through it, so resolve to use it as an opportunity to organize, synthesize, and work with the body of preclinical knowledge you've learned in the past two years. Approaching the challenge with that mindset will make the process much more pleasant for you.

"My medical school allotted five weeks to study for Step 1," Adam recalls. "I spent six days a week in the library, about twelve hours a day or so. I also scheduled time to go to the gym to get my mind off of things."

If you're a D.O. student, you will be on the same path, but instead of the USMLE Step 1, 2, and 3, you will take the Comprehensive Osteopathic Medical Licensing Examination (COMLEX), which is also broken into three Step-like exams given in the same sequence. Some D.O. students ultimately elect to take both the USMLE and the COMLEX in order to keep their residency options open. See the AACOM Web site (www.aacom.org), the COMLEX Web site (www.nbome.org), or the appendix on page 271 for links to more information.

CONFRONTING FAILURE AT CHECKPOINT 1

We all have bad days, bad months, and extraneous circumstances that prevent us from performing to our highest potential. The Step 1 Exam, though, is a bad time to underperform. These scores *do* matter, and they *do* impact your ability to get the residency of your choice. So what do you do if things go wrong?

The first step in addressing a poor performance on the USMLE Step 1 Exam will be meeting with your dean to discuss a plan for how to proceed. If you failed the exam or have scores you deem to be unworkable, you should immediately start rescheduling another administration of the exam. Many schools require that you pass Step 1 before you can proceed to the third year of school, so you certainly don't want to be waiting to finish up your boards while your classmates are already in the wards. Meet with your dean, find out what your school's policy is, and be prepared to present to him/her with a plan of how and when you intend to remedy the situation. People *do* fail Step 1 and still go on to have productive careers in medicine. The test now is how you confront and remedy your failure.

The next critical step is figuring out what exactly happened. You need to be brutally honest with yourself here. Review your score report from the National Board of Medical Examiners (NBME) and look at the distribution of your individual subject scores. Were you exceedingly weak in certain areas but strong in most others, or were you somewhat weak across the board? Look back over your practice tests and review the progression of scores. Look for areas you didn't review or for evidence you weren't really honest with yourself when you thought you had mastered a subject area.

Finally, start the process all over again, but watch yourself closely. Don't allow yourself to blithely pass over wrong answers or pass off mistakes due to carelessness. Be disciplined! Dig deep, and muster the resolve and stamina to review carefully. Enlist the help of your friends or support network to help you restore your confidence and keep you on track. It will be critical with this second set of scores to prove to your future residency that you had a bad day but redoubled your efforts and came back from defeat to triumph.

The road to physicianhood goes through this checkpoint. You cannot get there without passing it, and you've come too far to turn back now.

Resolve to win!

PART FOUR

The Clinical Years

CHAPTER 16

Life on the Wards

Medicine is learned by the bedside and not in the classroom.
Let not your conceptions of disease come from words heard in the lecture room or
read from the book. See, and then reason and compare and control.
But see first.
—SIR WILLIAM OSLER

AT LAST, YOU'VE left the breakwater of second year behind and find yourself rolling in the open seas of the real world of medicine. Already, the endless hours in the library and looming exams seem a blur, shadows of another life best left behind. Ahead lies the consummate adventure—and challenge—of actual patients in the wards and clinics. You're about to discover what you've been waiting for.

Welcome to the wards!

Your schedule and your life will change dramatically as you enter the clinical phase of your training. The traditional September-to-May academic year will fall away, as will the arbitrary time constraints of quarters and semesters. Instead, your life on the wards will be governed by the sequence of your rotations and the service you're on.

At times, it will seem like you're forced to reinvent yourself every six weeks as you assume a new persona, a new knowledge base, and a new set of responsibilities. But at the end of it all you will have had an experience virtually unparalleled in education—the opportunity to try on literally every facet of your profession and reach an informed decision about which clinical field interests you the most—and will become your chosen specialty.

"I think the hardest part was often not knowing exactly what one's role should be," Carolyn notes. "In the preclinical classes, one is generally told what the student needs to do/read/study to prepare for the test and do well. On the wards, oftentimes no one tells the student what to do. I think that can be very unsettling."

ROTATIONS

Your third year starts in June or July of the summer after your second year, so say good-bye to summers off. But by now, Step 1 is a receding memory from the spring, and you will find yourself driven with anticipation. You will probably have a week to two weeks of transitional class work followed by your first rotation. The actual sequence of your third-year rotations (or "clerkships," as they are sometimes called) is given to you in the spring of your second year. Typically, you will first pass through a set of core, or required, rotations. Since only a few students can do a rotation at any one time, everyone's sequence of rotations will be somewhat different.

The classic core rotations include internal medicine, surgery, pediatrics, obstetrics and gynecology, and psychiatry. Many med schools now also require a rotation in emergency medicine, and some also require one in family medicine. The typical third-year rotation lasts six weeks, though individual rotations may vary. Vacations will be spaced out between rotations. You will usually work throughout the summer, have a week off in the fall, work until Christmas, have a standard Christmas break, then resume rotations in January with another week off in the spring.

WHAT YOU NEED TO LEARN FROM YOUR ROTATIONS

You will have two primary goals for each of your rotations. First, you want to develop a working knowledge of the fundamentals of each specialty. This will include a review of the relevant anatomy, physiology, and pathophysiology, a sense of the most common diagnoses and differentials, and familiarity with essential workups and basic management of patients on that service. You will be expected to be an active member of a team of students, residents, and attending physicians (faculty) seeing patients in clinics or caring for them on the wards. Second, with each rotation you will be expected to continue to refine your history-taking, physical-exam, diagnostic, and documentation skills. These are broad and universal skills, and each rotation will challenge you to refine these fundamental clinical tools and understand how they are applied by physicians in each specialty. You will be surprised by how differently each specialty views the elements of these basic skills. Over time, you will adopt and adapt elements from many different experiences and gradually develop your own practice style.

Many people feel frustrated in their first few rotations because the information they spent so many hours memorizing during the preclinical years doesn't seem applicable to the cases they're seeing in the wards. The truth is, what you need to know is all in your head, but it's organized differently. In the preclinical years, you were given a disease and expected to memorize all the details about it. On the wards, you will be presented with a patient who has a relatively nonspecific constellation of symptoms and be expected to deduce the disease from these clues. This is a wholly opposite way of thinking that will feel foreign at first but will grow easier and more comfortable with time.

Oh, and there's one more important thing:

While the ultimate goal is to craft you into a knowledgeable and effective clinician, people *do* realize that you're just starting out. In the beginning, you won't be expected to know everything about clinical medicine or about the field you are rotating through. You won't be expected to make direct life-and-death decisions about patient care without assistance and oversight. As you progress in your rotations and gain experience, you will be trusted with greater degrees of responsibility and independence.

Remember that these programs are closely supervised. You're not going to kill any patients with your decisions during a rotation.

A TYPICAL DAY ON THE WARDS

The experience you have on individual rotations will vary widely, but there are some general commonalities, particularly for your core hospital rotations. In the hospital, you typically will be divided into teams. Your team will most likely be composed of a single senior resident who oversees the team, one or two interns (first-year residents) who are responsible for the majority of patients on the service, and you. Initially, your role will be to assist an intern with the patients that he or she is responsible for. In your first rotation, you'll take one patient at a time. As you develop more experience and expertise, you will start carrying more and more patients, until ultimately you will start carrying patients on your own with oversight only from the senior resident or attending physician. This gradual ramping up of responsibility will be a common theme throughout the rest of your medical training.

Prerounds

Your day on the wards will usually start early—very early! With most inpatient (i.e., hospitalized) patients, you will be required to preround. This means that for all patients to whom you've been assigned, you will review their charts, note any events that occurred overnight or since you last saw them, gather any new laboratory information, and review any intervening test results or X-rays. You will interview and examine the patients daily. Finally, you will record your observations, findings, and an assessment and clinical plan in daily chart notes, and if you're smart you'll run your thoughts past your intern to ensure that you're on the right track.

Sound like a lot to accomplish? Wait until you have to do it on six to ten patients—you'll be expected to do that as a resident!

The good news is, as with most things, you'll get more comfortable with the process and become much more efficient over time. In the meantime you'll have to arrive early enough to get your notes written before your team rounds begin, sometime between 6:00 A.M. (on many surgery services) and 9:00 A.M. (on various other rotations). When you start out, you'll probably need to get to the hospital at 4:00 or 5:00 A.M. to complete your prerounds. Eventually, though, you'll figure out ways to optimize your data gathering and minimize these early hours.

"The hardest part about the transition to wards medicine was learning to multitask," Kate notes. "Seeing multiple patients while trying to move efficiently through each patient exam and write a clear and concise note just took practice."

Rounds

With your notes safely nestled into your patients' charts, and with another cup of hot coffee in hand, you're ready for the team rounds.

This is the first and primary time during the day that you will meet with the entire team and review your service. Most services do walk rounds, also known as "bedside rounds," during which you walk throughout the hospital visiting each patient on the service.

When the team comes to your patient, you will be expected to give a brief presentation on that patient's case. If it is a newly admitted patient, you will be required to present a complete history and physical exam, a diagnostic differential, and an assessment and plan. If it is a patient the team is already familiar with, you will just provide a review of the patient's presentation of symptoms, an update on overnight events, and a review of the day's labs and your physical findings. Finally, you will present an overall assessment of the patient's condition and a plan for each item on the patient's problem list.

Your attending physician and senior resident will then ask you questions about the patient and the pathophysiology of the patient's condition. This Socratic exchange between you and your superiors on the team is known as "pimping"—a daily cold-call on your medical knowledge base that is designed to expose and fill in any gaps in your understanding. Since you know this is coming, you should research each of your patients' presentations to aid you in reaching an informed diagnosis.

The best attendings will take these opportunities to teach and lead you to a better understanding of the diagnostic process and an effective treatment plan. Some attendings will, admittedly, be less forgiving and less gentle. Either way, you will learn immensely from the process.

"Know your patients well—talk to them, learn about their symptoms and also about what they are like as people," Carolyn advises. "Read about their diseases, understand what medicines they're on and why. Practice your presentations so you learn how to present succinctly only the pertinent positives and negatives. Read about one topic (even if only a few pages) every day. Always be willing to help. Help your fellow classmates—being competitive with them is not pleasant and doesn't look good."

At the end of your presentation you will make a list of the day's action items for that patient. Your team rounds will typically take several hours, meaning your first respite won't come until midmorning. This is when you will be expected to follow up on each of the action items on your patient, be it entering new orders for medications, following up on new tests, calling in consultations, or getting more history. You'll then grab a quick lunch on the run and jump into the afternoon.

Lectures

As your afternoon begins, you will typically have a one-to-two-hour lecture, usually given by the senior resident or the attending physician. These sessions will provide you with the bulk of the clinical teaching for the service you are on. During these lectures, you will review common complaints and disorders seen by that specialty and the most effective treatment programs for them.

Clinics

Later in the afternoon, depending on your rotation, you will also spend time in the outpatient clinics or in the operating room. If you're in the clinics, you will be expected to go in and see scheduled patients in exam rooms on your own. You will complete your history and physical, then come out and present the patient to a senior resident or attending physician. That person will then pop in and see the patient, confirm your findings, and pursue the agreed-upon course of treatment. This will be excellent practice because it forces you to work through individual cases and try to reach your own conclusions before discussing the case with a superior. Furthermore, these are the long-dreamed-about moments when you're alone in a room with a patient, and you *are* the physician.

"At first I was quite anxious around patients, and I suspect they were also anxious with me," Adam admits. "As I learned to project some confidence in my skills, I noticed my patients trusting me more. It is important to remember that patients are just people—they don't always expect you to know everything. The most important skill to master is compassion."

Call

You will also periodically take call with your team. If it's a call day, that means your team is responsible for admitting patients to the hospital on your service for a twenty-four-hour period. You will spend the night in the hospital and assist with the initial evaluation and management of patients. You will be responsible to follow any patients you personally admit for your team. These are often long nights of little (or no) sleep. But these will be some of the most memorable experiences you will have in your entire medical-school career. Whisking the patient with the ruptured appendix off to the OR at 3 A.M., or helping a terminal cancer patient find relief and peace from his pain in his last moments of life are sobering, meaningful, and deeply gratifying experiences. True, you will also find yourself admitting patients with intractable back pain or patients who are angry at their illness and who want to take it out on you, and, yes, the sleep deprivation can be hard to adjust to. But it is precisely these long hours that will bring an appreciation for the broad spectrum of illness, the immense body of medical knowledge amassed to treat illness, and the subtleties and nuances of patient relations.

This is what you went to med school for.

The logistics of call are fairly straightforward. While on call, you will usually wear scrubs provided by the hospital. The pager that you imagined as a badge of distinction and used to dream of wearing will become an incessant, nagging voice on your hip. You will eat with your team between patients or whenever you get a chance. There will be a call room available with a simple desk and bed for you to use to complete paperwork or to catch a few precious minutes of sleep when you get the chance.

After a call night, you will sign out to the other members of your team who weren't on call and go home, usually around noon the following day. You will be exhausted but also fulfilled. Your head will likely be filled with more questions than clarity. Suddenly, your reading will take on a dimension of urgency. Those subtle points you glossed over in the preclinical phase, those arcane details, will come back to you now as you see, touch, hear, and feel pathology in action. You'll then catch a few hours of sleep, and before you know it you will be back again, prerounding on your patients for the start of another day.

"Be a team player, and remember that your education is occurring in real time along with a sick patient's medical care," Adam says. "The patient comes first. Learning everything you can about your patient is the best education you can get on the wards."

Dealing with the Culture Shock

The transition to life in the wards may come as a bit of a shock. You're a long way from the preclinical classroom, and for some this may be your first foray into the professional world. As a preclinical student, you made your own schedule and worked fairly independently as you attended classes, studied, and took exams. On the wards, you will be expected to be an active member of a busy team that is caring for patients. If you fail to carry your weight, if you fail to follow up on tests or to put in orders as instructed, patient care will be compromised. You may feel very unsettled during your first few weeks in the wards, since your supervisors don't always tell you exactly what to do. If you find yourself lost, or wondering whether you ought to take some action, you should always ask.

If you are new to working on teams, or new to the professional environment, here are three quick but critical pointers to help you smooth the transition.

Professionalism

First, act professionally in all you do. In class you could get away with dressing in torn jeans and T-shirts; you could chew gum, make crass jokes, or show up a few minutes late. On the wards, you are endowed with the respect and responsibilities of a student-doctor, and it is imperative that you act the part. This means dressing neatly and professionally, and treating your patients, team members, and everyone in the hospital professionally and with respect.

Reliability

Second, be an active, responsible, and reliable team member. It is sometimes tempting just to shuffle through a rotation and do the minimum required—particularly if you already know the rotation is of limited long-term interest to you. But if you seek out opportunities to get actively involved, you will be impressed with the return on your investment. You'll find you get additional teaching, the more interesting patients, and perhaps even opportunities to try your hand at important procedures. Maintain a good attitude in all things you do, no matter what the hour. Try to anticipate your patient's and your resident's needs, and pave the way ahead for them. If you know the team is going to need to review the patient's old chest X-rays in light of a new finding, track those films down ahead of time. Most importantly, know your patients and be an advocate for them. Learn everything you can about them and their histories. Spend time talking with them and understanding their illnesses. Do your homework, research their conditions, the most common presentations, the key diagnostic criteria, the most common therapies, and the typical complications.

Be mindful, however, of the fine line between being an active, professional team member and being a suck-up. It's great to help out, but it's not okay to constantly try and prove how smart you are or to brownnose your attendings and residents. Your supervisors are busy people who are there primarily to take care of patients, to learn, and to teach. If you gum up the works with your pandering, grandstanding, or by copping an attitude, you will quickly find yourself isolated. And that's not where you want to be on the wards.

Humility

As in most professions, the best thing you can do as you enter the clinical world and start out in the unfamiliar terrain of the wards is to display humility. Be honest about the limitations of your knowledge and experience. A sincere "I don't know—can you teach me how to do that?" will go a long way.

No matter how hard you get pimped, no matter how stupid you feel, remember that your sole purpose on the wards is to learn as much as you can in order to become an experienced and well-rounded clinician.

The way to succeed in the clinical years is actually very simple:
- Be helpful to the team you are on without being a suck-up.
- Be knowledgeable about what you are supposed to know, and be honest when you have no idea what you are talking about.
- Be fun to work with without being flippant or disrespectful.
- Do not forget that you are paying extremely good money for the educational experience, and while a certain amount of scut work is the price you pay the team for your training, if you are not getting the education you need, you have to be vocal (albeit politically so) about getting it.

All of the people I know who had difficulties in their clinical years violated one or more of these key principles.

—Adam

How to Survive on the Wards

Although all of this seems overwhelming, you will quickly find yourself getting into the swing of the daily routine on the wards and even into the regular cycles of new rotations and new roles. The key thing to remember on the wards is to keep your head above water and to stay positive. You will have rotations you will like less than others. You will have long and stressful nights. There will be whole seas of clinical information you don't know, especially when you are put on the spot on rounds. Do everything you can to stay on top of your patients and keep up-to-date on your reading and studying.

Stay connected to your patients, and focus on learning all you can so that when you're out on your own, you can draw on these fundamental clinical experiences. Never lose sight of the fact that what to you is another long night of writing admission history and physicals (H & Ps) is to your patients a scary experience of being admitted to the hospital with an illness. Recognize what it is you get to do, appreciate your role in it, and be an advocate for your patients. In the end these are the things that will make all your clinical time gratifying and fulfilling, and make you eager to come back day after day.

"I can't remember half of what I learned in my preclinical years," Pete admits, "but I still can't encounter disease in the hospital without thinking back to the first patient who taught me about that particular disease, its differential, and its treatment."

Reading

Most students are thrilled to be free of the yoke of preclinical classes and out into the relevant world of real clinical medicine. This does not mean, however, that your hours of studying are behind you. You will still be expected to read and study for each rotation you do, and you must continue your vigilant preparation for your board exams.

The good news is that all your reading and studying will take on an edge of real urgency as you actually see the pathology in your patients. Suddenly you'll realize you don't understand the process of congestive heart failure as well as you thought you did, and the vague list of possible treatments you memorized as a second-year isn't coming to you as you admit a patient with the disease at 2 A.M.

"I don't think you can ever read too much, listen to a patient too much, or have too much on your differential diagnosis," Deb states.

There are references for you to read and study that will give you the information you need—and finding these sources is the key to studying in the last two years of medical school. Your emphasis now will turn from textbooks and basic science sources to focus on sources emphasizing clinical relevance. For each specialty under the sun there are basic clinical texts that present the fundamentals of that specialty. These are generally good, but they tend to be long and exhaustive and difficult to cover quickly in a few hours on a call night. They also tend to delve more deeply into reviewing the underlying pathology and pathophysiology that, as we mentioned, is not the focus of your current studies. Your goal here should be finding a source with just enough of a review of the disease process to jog your memory and much more information about diagnosis, treatment, and complications.

The reference books most commonly used by medical students are the brief, specialty-specific reviews. These have a range of titles that sound like *Essentials of Surgery* or *Essentials of Obstetrics and Gynecology*. Your best bet is to peruse the amazon.com Web site or your med school's bookstore and find one that appeals to you. The formats for these types of review books vary broadly, so pick one that you find intuitive and appealing and go with it. Most are arranged either as a topic-by-topic review or as a series of topic-oriented questions. This latter format lends itself well to being prepared for the tough pimp questions when you're in your fourth hour of holding the retractor in the OR and the surgeon asks you to name all the encapsulated organisms that pose particular risk to patients who have undergone a splenectomy (an actual pimp question that Dr. Bissell bombed . . . but you can rest assured he went home and read up on it!).

A reference should be made here to the generic clinical references as well. There are basic, fundamental skills and tasks that are universal to most specialties. Things like what orders need to be included in any basic admission or how to calculate a patient's ideal body weight for drug dosing. To this end, there are a large number of basic clinical reference texts designed to fit in your pocket and be frantically consulted when you're sitting in front of the computer admitting a patient. Again, formats vary widely, so it will be pretty much up to you to find one you find easy and concise. You will probably find these books very helpful during the first few rotations and then less frequently relied on as you develop more clinical acumen. (Consult the appendix on page 271 for a list of several of the most popular standard references.)

Finally, many students use the ubiquitous personal digital assistant (PDA) as their quick reference of choice. With today's technological advancements, you can pretty much hold an entire reference library in your hand. There is a seemingly infinite variety of tools, calculators, and programs for your education and entertainment. This is a constantly evolving arena, so you will do best to search the Internet and find out what's currently available and most popular. Many of the titles are available as free or low-cost shareware. Talk to your senior students and residents as well to solicit their informed opinions as to what they found to be most useful (again, see the appendix for a list of some of the most popular resources).

BASIC CLINICAL SKILLS

The Foundations of Doctoring course you took at some point during your first two years of med school should have given you some of the basic clinical skills you will now draw on in the wards. Many find, however, that this introduction seems paltry when faced with your first patient and your first real hospital admission. Don't panic! Use your handy pocket references and these pointers and you'll breeze your way through the first of many admissions.

Interviewing and physical-exam skills

It is normal to feel somewhat bewildered and befuddled as you get ready to approach your first patient. There are a couple of keys to making this encounter smoother. First, arm yourself with a checklist of what you need to accomplish. Your goal here is twofold: first, you need to get to know the patient, understand his or her condition, and begin thinking about treatment; second, you need to succinctly record all the pertinent data you collect into the patient's chart so that others can draw on your complete history and physical. So until taking an H & P gets to be automatic, you'll be wise to go into the room with a template document labeled with the key information you need to acquire. This list should include headings for:

- Chief complaint
- History of present illness
- Review of systems
- Medications
- Allergies
- Past medical history
- Past surgical history
- Family history
- Social history
- Physical exam

Second, spend time talking to patients before you examine them. This will allow you to develop a relationship with them and put them at greater ease. Strive to make it a conversation rather than an interrogation. Be friendly, conversational, and direct. Try to project confidence without being cocky. When you begin performing the actual exam, be methodical and cover all the bases. You will see your residents and attendings cutting corners and hitting only the high points of an exam, but at this stage you should err on the side of being more thorough.

Third, as you examine the patient, consider questions that you missed during your interview. Keep a running dialog during the exam. This will put your patient at ease and allow you to fill in any gaps left during the interview portion of your consult.

Making chart entries

Once you've completed your detailed interview and exam, it's time to record the data in the chart for everyone to see and refer to. As you write out your H & P, recall that the chart is both the primary means of communication among care providers as well as the very critical legal record of the patient's care. As such, all your entries should be clear, legible, concise, and professional.

Any chart entry should begin with the date and time and type of chart entry you are making. It should also include who is making the entry. Thus your H & P might read: "03/15 @ 2100—Admission H & P, Orange Team, (MSIV)." This tells everyone what kind of entry it is, what team it's going on, and who did the entry. Other chart entries you make will include:

- Daily progress notes
- Procedure notes
- Event notes
- Transfer or discharge summaries
- Discharge instructions

The proper format for each of these chart entries can be found in any of the reference books listed above. These entries will feel foreign at first but will quickly become a matter of routine.

Calling consultants and other services

One of your jobs as a medical student may be calling other services for consultations on your patient. This can be a daunting task since you are representing your service to another team or even another attending directly. Again, your approach here should be to be clear and concise. Instead of launching into the patient's entire medical history leading up to this admission, start the conversation by stating what it is you need: "I have a sixty-five-year-old woman who presented with a heart attack and now seems to be in renal failure. We would like to get a renal consult, please." Then, if further background is requested, you can launch into the specifics of the case. Better to give the consulting individual the relevant general principles of the case and save the details for specific questions. More than likely all they're looking for is the patient's name, room number, and basic problem. They'll uncover the rest for themselves as they review the chart and meet the patient.

Working with nurses and other team members

Part of the reason many of us went into medicine is because, well, you get to be "The Doctor." Let's face it, it's a bit of an ego trip. You know—the whole "God Complex" thing. It's both exhilarating and scary to be the final authority on something as important as someone's health care. What you'll quickly discover, however, is that health care is 100 percent a team sport. You cannot render care in a vacuum, and if you are so filled with hubris as to believe that only your opinion and insight matters, you will have a short and most unpleasant career in medicine.

You will be astounded by how much you have to learn from your health-care colleagues, and how wonderfully symbiotic your working relationship can be. Treat your team members with ultimate respect and be open to learning from them. Many, if not most, have been doing this for much longer than you have. Consider their perspective and insights.

KEEPING PERSPECTIVE AND DEVELOPING YOUR CLINICAL PERSONA

As with every stage of your medical training, it will be challenging at times to maintain your balance and perspective during your clinical rotations. In many ways, though, this is the most crucial time for you to keep your eye on the ball. Not only will you shortly be faced with deciding what specialty to pursue, your clinical grades and evaluations will also be a major factor in your residency application, especially in your core rotations. It's worth doing what it takes to keep yourself focused, excited, and on task.

One of the best things to do is to seek a mentor. As you go along, you may start to have some inkling of what specialties suit you. Consider seeking out a professor you particularly like, or an attending whose style resonated with you, and set up some time to talk with that person. Solicit that person's advice on how to become a competitive candidate for a residency in that field, and understand the path your mentor took to get to his or her present position. Mentorship needn't be a binding contract—you can just be curious and interested in gaining more information and insight. Most people respond very well to someone else showing interest in what they do, and they will go out of their way to discuss their field with you and arrange opportunities for you to get involved or get more exposure.

Along that same line, consider joining the local interest group for the specialty you're exploring. Most schools have organized groups dedicated to specific specialties. The groups meet periodically, coordinate extra learning opportunities, and may have intermittent guest speakers. It's great to get together with other students who are contemplating the same specialty to discuss the details.

No matter what field you are considering, be sure to closely observe the physicians around you and take mental notes on what makes a good doctor. Along the way, you will encounter fantastic physicians who are inspired and compassionate and intelligent. You may also meet some doctors who are bitter, burnt out, alcoholic, or even borderline incompetent. As you encounter this range of individuals, be sure to take note of the key characteristics that you would like to either emulate or avoid as you develop. Imagine the kind of physician you want to be, and take the time to recognize that your experiences and observations right now are actively shaping your own clinical persona.

Finally, if you need a shot of enthusiasm, begin thinking about residency. Pick a field you think you might be interested in and start doing some research. Skip ahead in this book to the sections on picking a specialty and doing residency research to get ideas about resources to draw on. Start perusing the Web pages of various residencies to get a feel for how the system works and what the different programs are like. This will not only serve as valuable education for the very near future when you begin to apply, but it will also make tangible the fact that you will eventually get out of medical school and on to the next level of your training.

BUT FOR NOW, IT'S STILL SCHOOL: REPORTS, GRADES, AND EVALUATIONS

No matter how refreshing it feels to be out of the classroom and into the clinics and wards, you're still in school, and the work you do will still be evaluated and end up on a transcript. In many ways, your clinical grades and evaluations will be *more* crucial for your residency application. Most residencies consider the preclinical years to be an important rite of passage, and your success therein rightly or wrongly judged by the USMLE Step 1 Exam. With the Step 1 Exam to handle the didactic portion of medical school, most residency programs tend to focus on the student's clinical performance as a measure of how well that student will perform as a resident.

In other words, this is your time to shine.

What can you do to optimize your performance? If you follow the strategies outlined above for surviving and thriving in the wards you should be well on your way to getting solid evaluations. This is key, since you will select several of these clinical evaluators to write your letters of recommendation for your residency application.

The actual transcript grade you receive is a little bit tougher to summarize. Some rotations will grade you almost solely on your clinical performance and your presentations. You may be expected to write up a few H & Ps, each a detailed history and physical with an academic differential and a discussion of the problem in the form of a minipaper, usually about two to three pages in length. Many rotations may also require you to take their service exam at the end of the rotation. This is a comprehensive exam produced by the specialty board. The residents may periodically take versions of this exam. They are typically quite hard and broad in scope. The best way to prepare for them is conscientious reading throughout the rotation and a solid specialty-review book designed for medical students. You may be able to track down practice tests, either through fellow students who have already completed the rotation or through your medical-school or university bookstore. Talk to residents to determine what is available at your school.

Overall, one of your best resources for how to survive and thrive in any given rotation will be your classmates who have gone before you. Since each of you will be on your own individual sequence of rotations, there will always be people in your class who have come before you and can give you an insider's view. Naturally, you have to take anyone's opinion with a grain of salt, since you may have different skills and weaknesses and thus perform differently in a given rotation. However, these survivors can be an invaluable guide to the lay of the land, to the best attendings and residents, and to the most useful reference resources. Use these people liberally to gather information.

"Unfortunately, I think how you are evaluated on clinical rotations sometimes has more to do with how well your evaluator likes you than how well you perform," Chris explains. "This is often influenced by what specialty you are going into. Many would agree that if you seem more eager to go into surgery, your surgeon evaluators are more likely to give you a higher grade than those who work just as hard but have communicated a decision about pursuing a different field. Ideally this should have nothing to do with your grade, but the reality is that from time to time, it does."

CHAPTER 17

Problems in the Wards—and
How to Deal with Them

Some minds are like concrete—all mixed up and permanently set.
—UNKNOWN

WE HOPE YOU'LL sail through your clinical years. Most people
find that they really enjoy their clinical rotations and that by
the time the fourth year rolls around, making a choice of specialty is
surprisingly hard. With that said, some rotations will be inherently
less appealing to you, and you may also find that you're simply less
suited to some fields than others. Medicine also attracts strong personalities, and you will likely encounter a person or two along the
way, often in the wards, with whom you do not mesh. This can make
for some uncomfortable moments or, if left unchecked, for some
career-limiting altercations. As such, this chapter aims to provide a
few simple suggestions for diffusing conflict in the stressful environment of the wards.

ACT WITH INTEGRITY

First and foremost, *always* act with integrity. This sounds simple
and self-explanatory but may be surprisingly challenging in practice. You will be pushed hard on many of your rotations, and cutting
corners, glossing over things, and deflecting responsibility or blame
for errors, either due to fatigue or out of fear of humiliation, will be
a powerful temptation. Furthermore, for the first time you will be
dealing with real patients who have complex personal and medical

issues. Many of your patients will be unpleasant, unsavory, and unclean. Some will come seeking narcotics and nothing more. Many will refuse to heed your advice or to come to terms with their illnesses. This will be frustrating and aggravating and will at times push you to the point of anger. Some of your attendings and residents may be abusive, angry, curt, unprofessional, uncaring, or downright negligent. Given the stressful nature of medical practice, you will also almost certainly encounter colleagues with personal and professional problems that they refuse to acknowledge or deal with.

So how, exactly, is one supposed to deal with all of this on top of everything else?

Make integrity your mainstay.

Treat everyone with respect. First and foremost, respect yourself. Stay focused on why you're there—to learn, to grow, and to help. Never let anyone infringe on your boundaries of decency and respect. If you feel these have been violated, excuse yourself, pull back, and regroup. Second, respect your patients. These are the people you're here to serve. Even those who are clearly seeking secondary gain or are lost in their own pathology deserve your attention and help. You may not be able to cure or even to help all your patients, but you can always treat them with respect and honesty. Finally, respect those who teach you. Be honest in your work and honest about your limitations. If you don't understand something, don't be afraid to say so. Work hard to address any deficiency or confusion, but never feel belittled. You are there to learn, and they are there to teach. It's as simple as that.

Respect your colleagues on your teams, support them in their struggles, and make sure you're carrying your load and are ready and willing to jump in when something needs doing. There's almost always more work than can be accomplished, so any given team member who doesn't carry his weight will be a further drag on your most precious resource—time.

Do everything in your power to make sure you are not that person.

RESOLVING CONFLICTS WITH
ATTENDING PHYSICIANS OR RESIDENTS

Even if you do all of these things and maintain the highest level of integrity, there *still* may be situations where conflicts arise. You may find yourself at odds with an attending or resident who, no matter how you approach a situation, escalates things, is consistently rude, offensive, or discriminatory, or refuses to teach you with the respect you deserve as a student.

Sometimes, it's as simple as a misperception that can be nipped in the bud and easily resolved. Sometimes, it's more than that—and when that happens, you must work hard to defuse such issues on the ward.

Your first approach to resolving such a conflict should be a simple, direct, and honest conversation with the individual. Try to initiate the discussion in a private and nonconfrontational way. Ask the person what it is that upsets them about the way you conduct yourself and for things you can do to improve the situation. Taking this approach can be disarming and can go a long way. Make the person feel listened to. Sometimes your efforts may span several conversations. Be sure to try to implement any reasonable suggestions the person offers to you.

Only after this initial approach fails should you take your concerns to the next level. If your problem is with a team member, go to your attending or senior resident. If it is with an attending, go to the department medical-student coordinator or to your dean. Again, your approach with each of these people should be measured, professional, and nonconfrontational. Be sure to clearly communicate that you tried to resolve the situation directly with the individual involved. Underscore that your goal is to resolve the situation and to optimize your experience on the rotation. Your concerns should be taken seriously and addressed by those in charge.

Understand, however, that by taking the conflict to a superior, you do risk escalating the tension between you and the individual or alienating him or her altogether, and drawing negative attention to yourself as well. Everyone on the wards is busy putting patient care first, and no one wants to have to take time out to resolve petty or unnecessary conflicts. As the old adage goes, "If you try to fight a skunk, you're going to end up smelling bad."

Unless the problem involves a truly serious offense like sexual harassment, racism, or bigotry, think carefully before you choose to escalate a conflict on the wards.

If you have particular concerns about how a rotation is going, or if it is a rotation that is especially important to you, it may be worth asking for a midrotation evaluation. This will usually just be an informal verbal review of your progress thus far. A good tactic is to approach your attending and say, "I'm really interested in doing well on this rotation. Can you give me some feedback on how I'm doing or what I could be doing better?" This emphasizes that you're eager to improve and will give you some specific areas in which to demonstrate improvement and proficiency. This approach will also help prevent you from being ambushed by a poor evaluation at the very end of a rotation you thought was going well.

If you do get ambushed despite this approach, or are otherwise justifiably dissatisfied with a grade or an evaluation, make an appointment to see the attending in charge of the rotation and discuss the situation. Hopefully you can come to terms and shed light on where that evaluator thought your performance was lacking. If it was misperception or miscommunication, talk it through and request to have the evaluation changed.

CHAPTER 18

Core Clinical Rotations

To study the phenomena of disease without books is to sail an uncharted sea,
while to study books without patients is not to go to sea at all.
—SIR WILLIAM OSLER

THIS CHAPTER WILL provide a brief overview of the core clinical rotations. Although there will be significant variability from school to school in the structure and schedule of these rotations, the rotations are fairly universal because they provide the fundamental experiences that will form the foundation of your clinical skills. Heed their lessons, and learn the basics well. Mastery of these skills will allow you to shine in the important elective rotations in your fourth year and will become a cornerstone of your practice.

INTERNAL MEDICINE

Your rotation in internal medicine will be a wellspring of these core skills. This is bread-and-butter stuff. The differentials are broad and the problems often complex. Despite having spent countless hours reading and memorizing the intricacies of human disease, you will be shocked to discover actual pathology before your eyes. Suddenly the clinical relevance of all your toils will snap into focus, and you will curse yourself for not paying better attention as you struggle to recall the details of a given condition.

Don't worry, this is normal.

All medicine is about pattern recognition. The first time you see a condition, its pattern may be subtle and your eyes, ears, and hands not well tuned. The second time you see it, a light may go on as you recognize signs and symptoms. By the third time, you will be surprised to find diagnoses screaming at you from the earliest encounter with a patient. It is tremendously exciting and rewarding to be able to say, "I know what you have, and I know what we can do to treat it."

Of course, not all your cases will be straightforward.

Disease can be subtle in its earliest stages, and presentations can be highly variable. This is where you need to develop strong clinical detective skills. You will watch your residents and attendings be equally baffled by patients and their presentations, and you will watch them systematically develop a list of differential diagnoses. Together you will step through this list sequentially and logically, evaluating the possibilities and ordering tests to confirm or exclude various things on the list. You will track the patient's progress, his exam, his lab and test results, and slowly bring the patient's picture into focus. You will target your therapies at symptoms, prioritized to address the most dangerous items on the differential list that you must act to protect that patient from immediately. Despite the eons of accumulated wisdom and all the sophistication of modern medicine, you will still encounter cases where no one knows for sure what happened to a patient, only that the person got better or died.

Medicine will forever be a humbling profession.

The basic routine of your rotation in internal medicine is largely described by a basic day on the wards. You may also have time in the outpatient or ambulatory clinic weekly or even daily. This will be a very different experience from the wards, more akin to your early patient experiences in the preclinical years. Most people find clinic somewhat frustrating because you don't know any of the patients personally and only have a few moments before seeing them to review their chart records and get up to speed on their care to date. Nonetheless, clinic is a good time to understand the differences in ambulatory and hospitalized pathology and to differentiate between patients you safely manage on outpatient status and those you need to admit for stabilization, testing, or comfort. This is also a time to observe your attendings as they interact with established patients with whom they have longitudinal relationships. These longstanding relationships are a major reason many people choose primary care as their field.

Career considerations—internal medicine

Most people who go into internal medicine as a career enjoy its differentials and the broad spectrum of patients that they see and care for. Because internal medicine is an adult specialty, your practice will be more limited in ages than the even broader specialty of family practice. The vast majority of internal medicine physicians, commonly called "internists," are in private practice. This usually means they have joined a group of other internists to form a basic office practice. They see their patients primarily in the office, and if those patients need to be admitted to the hospital, they will care for them throughout their hospital stays. Internists will usually share call with the other partners in their practice. Call duties will include responding to telephone questions throughout the night and going in to the ER to see any patients from the practice who need admission.

Your options for subspecialization in internal medicine are extremely broad. After completing a basic residency in internal medicine, you can complete an approved fellowship. The range of possible fellowships in internal medicine includes adolescent medicine, allergy and immunology, cardiology, endocrinology, gastroenterology, geriatrics, hematology, infectious disease, nephrology, oncology, pulmonology and critical care, rheumatology, and sports medicine. Subspecialists obviously have a much more narrowly defined scope of practice. Many of these also focus on a variety of specific procedures, such as cardiac catheterizations, colonoscopies, or dialysis. Similar to primary-care internists, these subspecialists tend to divide their practice between clinic time and hospital time. The income potential for the subspecialists who focus on procedures is generally considerably higher than that of primary-care internists.

An additional option in internal medicine that is growing in popularity is the hospitalist. These are physicians who solely admit and care for patients in the hospital. Many primary-care internists will contract with hospitalists to handle all their admissions and inpatient care. This frees primary-care doctors to focus on their office practice and reduces their after-hours workload considerably. The hospitalists, in turn, don't have to worry about an office practice, and they have the luxury of essentially working shifts, eliminating the need for regular call.

"I always loved the holistic nature of internal medicine as well as the academic side of it," Adam recalls. "Internists apply an intellectual approach to patient care that I find very intriguing."

"I found that what I most enjoyed in all my clerkships were the internal medicine–related aspects of each rotation," Carolyn explains, "like the management of patients with respiratory, cardiovascular, and neurologic illness during my rotation in the surgical intensive care unit; the pathobiology of malignancies in gynecologic oncology; medical issues in high-risk obstetrics; and the evaluation of altered mental status in psychiatry. I felt like I learned the most on my internal-medicine rotations, and I was attracted to medicine because of its constant intellectual challenge."

PEDIATRICS

The first thing they'll tell you on your pediatrics rotations is, "They're *not* just little adults." And it's true that since most of medicine is geared toward the adult patient, it takes some time to adjust your thinking to encompass the physiologic and developmental considerations of caring for peds patients. Suddenly all your drug dosages are in milligrams per kilogram, and your IV fluids have to be half their normal concentration. You quickly realize that taking a useful history from a four-year-old is tough and requires a lot of interpretation. Often too late, you discover that sick kids can be subtle and that they tend to look okay right up until the point they crash. Finally, you will lose your breath over the strength, composure, and attitude of kids with chronic and terminal illnesses. There is much we can learn from them, both as physicians and humans.

On the other hand, kids also tend to be healthy, don't generally have self-destructive behaviors, and if they are sick they tend to get better. This is incredibly refreshing after you've spent six weeks caring for chronic alcoholics, obese hyperlipidemics recovering from their third heart attack, and lung-cancer patients who are still smoking and insist it has nothing to do with their disease. It's gratifying to be able to soothe scared kids, to be able to explain an illness to the child and the family, and to help the little ones get better because of the therapies you instituted.

There is something of a cultural schism between the adult medical world and the pediatric medical world. If you've already done a series of adult rotations, be prepared to adopt the "peds view" for the next several weeks. Be sure to read the first few chapters of your review book of choice on how to approach the peds patient before you start the rotation. Keep at hand a good reference for drug dosages and common peds illnesses. Read in your spare time about the important differences between adult and pediatric versions of even common illnesses like diabetes. Immerse yourself in the peds world and, as with all rotations, you will grow and learn at a dramatic rate.

Your peds rotation will follow a similar structure to that of your internal-medicine rotation. The bulk of your time will be spent on inpatient pediatric care, with a smaller portion going to clinic and various pediatric subspecialties. Try to make sure you cover a complete range of ages from neonatal through adolescent. Unfortunately this probably means you won't spend enough time in any one area or age group to gain real comfort, but remember—your goal here is to survey the specialty. If you choose to specialize in pediatrics, you'll have your entire residency to intensely study each age; if you're going into something else, you'll be well served by appreciating the very different diseases and needs of kids of all different ages.

Career considerations—pediatrics

Much like internal medicine, the bulk of pediatrics is practiced by primary-care pediatricians from their offices. Since kids less frequently require hospitalization, the majority of pediatric illnesses are managed on an outpatient basis. Unfortunately, since kids require less direct care and fewer procedures, the reimbursements from insurance and Medicaid are lower, and therefore pediatrics is historically one of the lower-compensated specialties. However, this shouldn't dissuade you if your passion is taking care of the little ones, as the payoff comes in many ways.

There are also a broad range of subspecialties in pediatrics that mirror those in adult medicine. These include adolescent medicine, allergy and immunology, cardiology, critical care, emergency medicine, endocrinology, gastroenterology, genetics, hematology and oncology, infectious disease, neonatology, nephrology, neurology, and pulmonology. It should be noted that several of the pediatric subspecialties can be entered either by completing a general peds residency and then a peds fellowship or by completing a specialty-specific residency and then completing a peds-specific fellowship. Thus, training in pediatric emergency medicine can be achieved either via a peds residency and peds–emergency medicine fellowship, or via an emergency medicine residency with a peds–emergency medicine fellowship. Similarly, to become a pediatric surgeon you must complete a standard general-surgery residency and then go on to a pediatric-surgery fellowship. The pediatrics residency is three years, and most fellowships are one to three additional years.

If you're considering pediatrics, you may feel frustrated by how many nonpediatric rotations you have to do.

Don't be.

While peds aren't little adults, there is much of adult medicine that applies to pediatrics, so any and all exposure will be helpful. Furthermore, many of the specialties you'll rotate through will include pediatrics in their demographics. If you're interested in peds, make sure you let this be known, and try to tailor your rotation to give you extra exposure to the pediatric patients of that specialty. Thus, by way of example, on your family-medicine clerkship you should request to spend more time on their newborn service, or while on surgery you should request to do a special week of pediatric surgery.

SURGERY

The lore of medical training is filled with horror stories of surgeons and surgical training. Medical students typically either dread or eagerly anticipate their surgery rotation, but either way they know it will be one of their most challenging and most memorable.

The surgeon's day is long, and he usually gets a very early start (often doing initial walking rounds at 6:00 A.M. and prerounds even earlier). Surgeons are classically quick, decisive physicians who pride themselves on their intimate knowledge of anatomy, disease, and complex surgical techniques. They consider themselves experts not just of the physical act of surgery but of care for the critically ill.

Interestingly, old surgical adages like "It takes steel to heal" or "You've got to cut to cure" reveal in part why surgery is such a high-intensity specialty and, concomitantly, such an intense rotation. While all physicians assume risk and responsibility as they prescribe therapies to their patients, nowhere is this risk more personal or apparent than in surgery. It's one thing to misdose a medication or delay a diagnosis, it's quite another to have personally opened up someone's belly, knicked a bowel or blood vessel, and caused a potentially catastrophic complication with your own hands. The weight of responsibility rests heavy on the surgeon's shoulders. They are able to achieve dramatic and rapid healing, but the complications that arise in their practices are often catastrophic.

Surgery is a tremendously broad field, so your rotation in general surgery will be only a fundamental introduction. Staying organized and being efficient are the keys to your surgical rotation. The service will tend to be busy and turn over fairly rapidly, so you will have to help to keep patients moving through. If you've just done other internal-medicine rotations, you may be accustomed to a more methodical, slower pace. You'll be surprised by how focused a surgeon's notes are. Surgeons are most interested in the problem at hand and the patient's historical and pathophysiologic context. They are less interested in an entire health history or major long-term preventative health strategies.

You should get some instruction on basic surgical techniques during your rotation. You won't need to learn how to do operations, but you will be expected to know how to tie proper surgical knots, how to suture, and how to assist during procedures. Your time in the OR will be spent mostly watching and holding retractors. In fact, you may find yourself contorted into uncomfortable positions for exceedingly long periods of time holding a retractor in an operative field that you can't even see from where you're standing. The good news is that if you're upbeat and eager, your efforts will get repaid with an invitation to close (i.e., close the incision with sutures and staples) or assist in more interesting ways on minor cases. Either way you will get to witness one of the most awesome sights in medicine— human anatomy in action. You'll discover the vivid beating body lying open before you is a far cry from your Human Anatomy corpse. You'll witness the dramatic impact of actual pathology on the body as you excise and repair disease. Finally, you'll be astounded at the elegant and complex techniques that have been developed to address the spectrum of surgical problems in human medicine. At the end of the rotation you will appreciate why a surgeon's training is so long and hard.

Career considerations—surgery

It has been said that the only reason to go into surgery is because you literally cannot imagine doing anything else in your life. The path of surgical training is arduous, and the realities of your professional practice after training aren't any easier. It is true that in this era of work-hour restrictions, surgical residents' lives have become more palatable. However, these restrictions have also made it more difficult to acquire the body of knowledge and to attain the level of procedural experience required.

A general-surgery residency is typically five years in duration. This will prepare you to do common surgical procedures throughout much of the body, focusing on the abdomen and soft tissues of the extremities. There are myriad surgical subspecialties from neurosurgery to urology. Most of the subspecialties start after your second or third year of general-surgery residency, though some, like plastic surgery and pediatric surgery, require you to complete your general-surgery residency before starting the fellowship.

Some surgeons are among the best-paid physicians in practice. The higher the level of training and the more complex the procedures, the higher the level of insurance reimbursement and, hence, the higher the salary. Neurosurgeons who spend seven or more years in training are among the highest paid. But to get there, you also have to commit seven years to living on a resident's salary. This means forestalling family, free time, and repayment of debt for that many *more* years.

If you believe you're interested in pursuing surgery, be sure to be appropriately vocal about it with your attendings and demonstrate it in your dedication to the rotation. This eagerness will likely open doors to more experiences for you. As you go through the rotation, examine closely the lives of your surgical colleagues. Can you see yourself doing what they do? Are they people that you want to spend a huge portion of your time with? Are you passionate enough about the subject matter and the opportunity to operate to dedicate yourself to the task—potentially at the cost of a personal life? If your answer is a resounding yes, then you will likely find the deepest rewards possible in your career.

"I came to realize about halfway through my required clinical rotations that I enjoyed being in the OR more than I enjoyed being on the wards," Deb admits. "This really became apparent one time in the OR while I was on my neurology rotation. One of the residents remarked that I seemed much more upbeat than I did when I was on the floor. I realized he was right. I liked the focused one-on-one patient care—trying to remember who out of fifteen patients on the floor had a creatinine of 1.2 just wasn't for me."

Ob/Gyn

Obstetrics and gynecology is a unique specialty in that it encompasses everything from primary care to surgery. As opposed to the horizontal organization of internal medicine, which cares for all genders and all adult ages with a wide array of problems, ob/gyn takes a vertical approach and cares solely for women and their unique health issues. It is true that the focus of ob/gyn care is on pregnancy, fertility, and gynecologic problems. However, the necessity of an annual exam means many women turn to their ob/gyn for the majority of their primary care. This includes routine health maintenance as well as management of some chronic conditions like hypertension or diabetes. Most ob/gyns will, however, refer their patients to an internist for more complex nongynecologic medical issues that go beyond their training.

The obstetrics portion of ob/gyn is focused on fertility, management of normal and abnormal pregnancies, and delivery of babies. On the gynecology side, ob/gyn physicians manage female hormone cycles, contraception, sexually transmitted diseases and other infections of the pelvis, gynecologic cancers, urinary complications, and all sorts of other pelvic disorders. This may sound like a lot to take in, and it is, but you will probably be surprised by how focused this specialty actually is, and how narrow the differentials often are. Ob/gyns have chosen a complex arena of anatomy and physiology, but they've developed a logical and highly structured approach to it that makes it comprehensible.

Your rotation in ob/gyn will be most similar to your surgery rotation. Like surgery, the service can be large and tends to turn over quickly. Your time will likely be divided between the ob side and the gyn side. During your ob weeks, you will start early and preround on the newly delivered postpartum patients. Your exam and notes will be strictly focused on complications associated with the delivery, making your rounds and note writing particularly quick. After you've seen your patients, you'll have quick work rounds with the senior ob resident and review the service. Many patients will be ready for discharge that day, so you will likely help prepare discharge instructions and get people ready to go. From there you will either go to the ob clinic and begin seeing women for outpatient pre- and postnatal care or you will go to the labor deck and help with deliveries. The clinic time will be pretty typical for most clinic work, but again you will be focused specifically on their obstetric history and current pregnancy.

Your time on the labor deck will be some of the most exciting experiences you'll have in medical school. You will primarily assist with vaginal deliveries, and by the end of your rotation you will likely be doing these almost completely without assistance (though an attending or a resident will be in the room with you). While it's generally a fairly straightforward procedure (remember women have been birthing babies at home without a doctor's help for centuries), it is nonetheless tremendously exciting and a great honor to be there and be able to help out. Furthermore, not every delivery goes smoothly, so you will also assist your team in complicated vaginal deliveries and emergent or scheduled cesarean sections in the adjacent OR.

During the gynecologic portion of your rotation, you will also divide your time between clinic and the wards, this time spending a much greater portion of your day in the OR. You will see everything from common infections to dysfunctional uterine bleeding to severe gynecologic cancers. Your clinic time will be spent with mostly pre- and postop patients. Your OR time will be spent assisting with various pelvic surgeries. Unfortunately the pelvis is a very difficult place to access surgically, so many of the procedures are done transvaginally (e.g., a transvaginal hysterectomy) or via minimal low abdominal incisions done in narrow spaces with minimal exposure. You'll have an attending and a senior resident already hunched over the small space being held open by your retractor, so your chances of getting a really clear view of the proceedings are fairly slim.

Many people have strong reactions to their ob/gyn rotation—they either love it or they hate it. Some are fascinated by the pathology, by the anatomy, and by the awesome process of giving birth. Others find the field too focused, get tired of doing so many pelvic exams, and find the surgery tedious. It will be a rotation you work hard on, but likely one you get a sense of accomplishment from since you can more easily grasp the spectrum of pathology and feel at least somewhat knowledgeable when pimped on rounds.

Career considerations—ob/gyn

As discussed, ob/gyns tend to have busy surgical and obstetrical practices that involve fairly high volumes of patients. Because they perform a wide variety of procedures, they tend to be well reimbursed. However, their practice is also fraught with risk. Complications associated with childbirth remain among the most highly rewarded malpractice cases since they are almost inevitably tragic. This produces staggeringly high malpractice insurance premiums that are among the largest in medicine, which can take a huge cut out of the bottom line.

For most of the last century ob/gyn, like every other field of medicine, was dominated by men. The last twenty to thirty years, however, has seen a reversal of that trend and a swing toward a predominance of women entering obstetrics and gynecology. While some female patients feel a woman practitioner may be more in tune with their needs and problems, others are more comfortable with a male physician, and still others don't care either way. It is true, however, that many male ob/gyn graduates are reporting increasing challenges in finding positions with an existing practice. As this is an emerging trend, if you are a male med student looking for placement in an ob/gyn practice, it is probably best to discuss strategy with your chief resident or attending.

The life of the ob/gyn doc is an arduous one, more akin to that of a surgeon. Most babies seem to be born in the wee hours of the morning, not conveniently at 3:30 in the afternoon (after you're done seeing your clinic patients). And, like their general-surgery colleagues, the complications of their procedures, both obstetrical and gynecologic, can carry a heavy toll. Nonetheless, most ob/gyns find their work tremendously rewarding and really enjoy the spectrum of diseases they see and the ability to spread their time between pure clinical medicine and the OR.

EMERGENCY MEDICINE

Emergency medicine is a relatively new field. As such, it has recently entered the mainstream and is only now becoming a required rotation at many medical schools. Emergency care was traditionally provided by internists, surgeons, pediatricians, and family-practice doctors, and the ER was just a place you either staffed occasionally to handle walk-ins or a place where you met your patients when you were going to admit them. Doctors in the ER were there either because they were required to be or because, for whatever reason, they had no independent practice of their own. With the advent of emergency medical systems in the 1960s, the modern ER began to take shape, and a few people found themselves drawn to the field as an independent specialty. Those initial heretics are now the forefathers (and foremothers) of the field, and the specialty is now a cornerstone of medical care in any community.

Today, the ER is not just where the majority of acute care is provided, it is also the portal to the entire hospital. ER physicians pride themselves on being able to care for any patient with any condition at any time—and as such, they are true generalists, with expertise a mile wide and an inch deep. Furthermore, most ERs see a tremendous volume of patients, both the critically ill and those with minor ambulatory complaints. As such, emergency medicine is always busy, varied, and fast-paced.

No matter what field you're going into, an ER rotation is a great opportunity to hone your general medical and surgical skills. You will get to do a bit of everything during your rotation and be afforded a degree of independence you may not get on other rotations. You will see patients, present their cases to a senior resident or attending, and then formulate a plan for their care. You will do almost all your own wound closures, splinting, and other minor procedures. You will order all the labs and ultimately help decide on the disposition of the patient. You will speak directly with consultants and admitting physicians. You will be an advocate for your patients and their needs. While you probably won't be directly involved in the critical-care aspects of emergency medicine, time permitting, you'll be invited into the resuscitation rooms to observe and sometimes help out with cardiac arrests, trauma victims, and other critically ill patients. With luck you might even get the chance to intubate a patient or start a central line.

Emergency medicine is a twenty-four-hour service, organized around shifts. You will work regular shifts just like your resident and attendings, usually eight to ten hours in duration. Your shift mix will likely involved day shifts (roughly 7:00 A.M. to around 4:00 P.M.), evening shifts (3:00 P.M. to 12:00 A.M.), and overnight shifts (11:00 P.M. to 8:00 A.M.). Depending on the size and volume of your ER, you may be assigned to rotate through various sections, like trauma, pediatrics, and ambulatory care. There will be regular didactics for medical students that focus on key areas of basic emergency medicine. In addition you will probably also attend the regular service conferences, as you do on any other rotation.

Career considerations—emergency medicine

Emergency medicine is fast-paced and relatively chaotic. To survive and thrive in this field, you have to like juggling a heavy patient load and you have to be eager to see the widest possible spectrum of pathology. One of the things that attracts people to emergency medicine is that sense of being able to care for any person at any time, with any condition. From day to day you never know what you'll end up seeing. While you won't know all the answers because you can't possibly master every field of medicine, you will be an expert at stabilizing sick patients with life-saving measures, diagnosing most medical and traumatic conditions, and getting the patients the long-term care they require either through inpatient admission with appropriate consultation or by arranging outpatient follow-up.

Another attractive aspect of emergency medicine is the lifestyle. Not only is it a well-paid specialty, it also has the fewest hours of almost any field. Most emergency physicians work anywhere from 120 to 140 hours per month clinically, half what many of their colleagues in other fields work. Furthermore, those hours are distributed over the range of shifts, meaning that ER docs often get to be at home with their families or out enjoying life while their colleagues are working regular daytime hours. The downside is that you will end up working a fair number of evenings and weekends, times when your physician colleagues from other fields and other professional friends will traditionally have off. As with most things, this is a trade-off that you need to evaluate for its fit with your own wants and needs in a career.

The most prevalent critique of emergency medicine is the lack of long-term continuity of care. While most ERs have their "frequent fliers," you'll rarely see the same patients on a regular basis. With that said, you have an opportunity to form a profound, albeit brief, relationship with the patients at an often very critical juncture in their lives. Some people prefer not to handle the critical-care aspects of the field or are turned off by the unsavory characters you often end up treating in the ER. You will see a tremendous amount of self-induced pathology, and the stories and circumstances of your patients' lives can be tragic and frustrating.

PSYCHIATRY

Psychiatry is another one of those rotations people either love or loathe. It is a definite departure from the majority of your clinical rotations. Your time will be spent observing and interviewing psychiatric inpatients and outpatients. You will learn the basic structure of the *Diagnostic Statistical Manual* (DSM), which is the psychiatrists' catalogue of disorders and their specific diagnostic criteria. You will discuss and write fairly extensive H & Ps that detail your impressions of the patient's condition and its origins. Finally, you will learn how to tailor therapies for different conditions based on both psychoanalytic as well as pharmacologic modalities. In addition to the strictly psychiatric patients, you may have the opportunity to participate in the inpatient consultation service. On this team, you will help evaluate medical and surgical inpatients with potential psychiatric issues like depression, dementia, suicidal ideation, or even psychotic behavior.

Most students are either fascinated by interacting with the bruised or broken psyche or find the experience boring or bizarre. Whatever your feelings, you should take note of the fundamental principles here. Almost any field you go into that deals directly with patients (pathology and radiology as the possible exceptions) will expose you to a diverse array of psychiatric issues, and as such this aspect of patient care will definitely impact your clinical practice no matter what specialty you choose.

Career considerations—psychiatry

The scope of mental-health care has evolved considerably in recent years. There are numerous midlevel providers such as psychologists and licensed clinical social workers who do a huge amount of the one-on-one therapy. Psychiatrists continue to play an important role in direct patient psychotherapy, but because of their highly specialized medical training they also tend to focus on medical management and more complex mental-health care. While the vast majority of psychiatrists are in a private-practice setting, there is a reemerging role for inpatient psychiatrists as psychiatric hospitalizations become shorter and more intense.

The psychiatrist has a range of subspecialization options. Fellowships include child and adolescent, geriatric, addiction, forensic, and research psychiatry. The psychiatry residency is three years long. Most fellowships are one year, with the exception of child and adolescent, which is three years long but can be combined with residency for a total of five years of postgraduate training. With fewer inpatient hospitalizations and almost no procedures, psychiatrists are among the lowest-paid physicians. However, their regular work hours and limited or nonexistent call make for an excellent lifestyle.

FAMILY MEDICINE

Your family-medicine rotation will be another broad-based experience during which you learn and improve a wide variety of fundamental skills. Family physicians, especially rural family physicians, literally see and do it all. Their demographics include newborns to geriatrics, and their skill set often includes obstetrics and basic surgery. In urban centers where there is a higher degree of specialized care available, the family physician may operate more like an internist and pediatrician combined, doing fundamental primary care and making appropriate referrals for subspecialty evaluations. In more rural settings, those resources are either wholly unavailable or at best difficult to access geographically. In these settings the family practitioner functions like the old-time country doctor—handling a broad range of issues independently, and in some cases even making house calls!

Your educational goals during this rotation will be to continue mastering the fundamental skills of patient interviews, exams, and evaluations. You will spend some time both in the clinics and on the wards. If you have the opportunity to do all or part of your rotation in a rural setting, take it. Even if you have no interest in family medicine or in rural medicine, you will experience an entirely different form of practice in the rural setting. First, you will probably be the only medical student for miles, so learning opportunities will abound. Furthermore, you will discover how spoiled we are to have every imaginable test and expert available to suit our every whim at the academic medical center we all grow up in clinically. It's very different when you're out there alone and the patient before you has something you don't recognize or something you will have a hard time treating. As the sole provider in an area, you also take on a unique and important role in the community, and you will form lasting relationships that are profoundly gratifying.

Career considerations—family medicine

Most family physicians will tell you they chose their field because they have the opportunity to be longitudinally involved in their patients' lives, caring for whole families or even generations of families and offering a consistent and trusted voice of advice and counsel on all things medical. Many family physicians now shy away from the obstetrics and surgical side of their practices for a variety of reasons, including liability concerns, the cost of insurance premiums, and because it is difficult to maintain true proficiency at those skills without everyday practice. However, as mentioned, the rural family doctor is still called on to do a little bit of everything.

Family physicians have a relatively rigorous schedule. As in other primary-care fields, their practices are generally orchestrated so that they attend to their regular clinic hours and then complete any admissions for the day and round on their hospital patients. The frequency of call nights will depend on the size of the group. If you're a rural family doc in solo practice, you're on every night, like it or not. Reimbursement varies considerably with the practice type and location but tends to be on a par with other primary-care specialties. There is an urgent need for rural primary care, so if you're drawn in this direction you'll likely find wide-ranging and attractive opportunities for some time to come.

"Family medicine was an obvious choice for me," Pete explains. "I knew I wanted service to communities to be a high priority in my professional life, and that I did not want to live in a major metropolitan area. I also saw that prevention is a far more pragmatic approach than treatment for the vast majority of disease affecting the United States today, and further that the emphasis on reactive health care today is doing our patients a disservice."

CHAPTER 19

Bringing It All Together Again:
The USMLE Step 2 Exam

One finger in the throat and one in the rectum makes a good diagnostician.
—SIR WILLIAM OSLER

JUST WHEN YOU thought you were free from the horrors of life in the library, that old beast the USMLE comes stalking you once more. Still wince every time you see a stack of flash cards? Still feel like *First Aid* for Step 1 is imprinted on your retinas like a solar flash? Well, the time has come to ramp up for the next board series exam.

Most schools require you to take the USMLE Step 2 Exam prior to graduation, and the best time to take it is between your third and fourth years, after you've just completed your core required rotations. The bad news is that Step 2 is a more rigorous test of your clinical knowledge and relies much more heavily on your clinical problem-solving skills than Step 1 did; the good news is that by the time they take it, most people find it significantly easier.

The Step 2 Exam is actually two separate tests: the Step 2 Clinical Knowledge (CK) Exam and the Step 2 Clinical Skills (CS) Exam. The CK Exam is a computerized multiple-choice exam in a format similar to the Step 1 Exam. Several years ago the folks who created the USMLE added the Clinical Skills Exam, in which students are observed interacting with simulated patients in a variety of scenarios and evaluated on their personal, professional, and technical skills.

Let's look at each of these components of the Step 2 Exam in closer detail.

The USMLE Step 2 Clinical Knowledge Exam

The goal of Step 2 is to provide a comprehensive review of basic clinical-medicine and physician skills. According to the USMLE, the test is structured in two conceptual sections; the first covers normal conditions and disease, and the second focuses on the four fundamental tasks of the clinician: promoting preventative medicine and health maintenance, understanding mechanisms of disease, establishing a diagnosis, and applying principles of management. As we've discussed, this test is almost 100 percent clinical in focus. The pathology and pathophysiology that is covered reflects the USMLE's high-impact disease list. This list includes common problems presenting commonly, less common problems where early detection or treatability are important considerations, and "noteworthy exemplars of pathophysiology."

The majority of your mentors used the First Aid series as a primary review text, supplementing those with other specialty-specific review books as needed. Most dedicated several weeks to studying, but often this was evening and weekend study time, not the 100 percent dedicated day-and-night kind of studying required for Step 1. Most of the information you will need should already be in your head from the rotations you just completed, so your study should be primarily to review and refresh the information.

Clinical information for all the specialty areas is weighted evenly on the test, even though the scope of information may vary significantly. Thus, even though internal medicine is a much broader, more comprehensive field, it will have the same number of questions as psychiatry. As such, time spent perfecting your knowledge of the more limited scope of psychiatric medications and therapies may make for a better overall score.

The written portion of the test is computer-based multiple-choice and lasts a full eight hours. It is administered at the Sylvan Prometric Testing Centers throughout the country. There is a wide range of dates when the test is offered, so you'll probably be most limited by whether the test center nearest you has an opening on the date you want. Register early if you plan on taking the test in an urban center or near your medical school—these test sites typically fill up well in advance.

THE USMLE STEP 2 CLINICAL SKILLS EXAM

At various points in the book, we've alluded to the fact that the USMLE now incorporates an examination of your clinical skills as well as your cognitive skills. In the late 1990s, the Objective Structured Clinical Examination emerged from the simulated-patient interaction efforts of various medical schools across the country. Schools recognized that students were learning their core clinical skills on real patients after they hit the wards, and that this often produced less-than-ideal patient encounters and incomplete skill sets. As a result, schools began using simulated patients (i.e., actors) to provide an opportunity for demonstrating fundamental interview and physical-exam skills. Instruction changed from simply what a physician needs to know to *how* he or she actually performs on the job.

The next logical step to these simulated encounters and lectures was to turn them around and use them as an evaluation tool to prove fundamental clinical competence in core skill sets. It didn't take long before the USMLE hopped on this bandwagon and realized that this clinical-examination component should be incorporated into the USMLE test regimen—and hence, the emergence of the USMLE Clinical Skills Exam.

The format of the exam is essentially a series of clinical encounters. It will seem as though you're seeing a series of patients in an office outpatient clinic. On exam day, you'll show up at the testing site and go through the registration process. You'll be given a sequence of patients to see at regular time intervals. At the start of the encounter you will be provided with a basic chart entry not unlike the one's you'd receive from your office staff. This will usually include the patient's chief complaint, vital signs, and possibly some background information. You will then be expected to enter the room, introduce yourself to the patient, carefully wash your hands, interview and examine the patient, discuss and formulate a plan for the patient, and then exit the room. On the outside you will have a few minutes to write a brief chart note about the encounter. Then you will move on to the next patient.

The USMLE has broken down the clinical encounter into three subcomponents for evaluation. The first subcomponent is the Integrated Clinical Encounter, which evaluates your ability to gather data and make a complete patient note. For the Communication and Interpersonal Skills subcomponent, you are expected to demonstrate your questioning skills and information-sharing skills while maintaining a consistent professional manner and establishing rapport. Finally, in the Spoken English Proficiency portion, you must demonstrate clear communication within the context of the doctor-patient relationship. This last portion is primarily intended for the international medical graduates who are attempting to achieve licensure in the United States.

Your Step 2 CS Exam will include eleven or twelve patient encounters. These include a very small number of nonscored patient encounters, which are added to pilot-test new cases and for other research purposes. Such cases are not counted in determining your score. The examination session lasts approximately eight hours, and two breaks are provided.

It's difficult to study effectively for the CS Exam, since it relies on a range of clinical skills that you will have developed over your first year on the wards. Many schools incorporate simulation training into their clinical rotations, so hopefully you'll be no stranger to working with simulated patients and playing the game. The USMLE Web site (www.usmle.org) includes tutorials, videos of encounters, and patient notes to practice on.

In general people from U.S. medical schools do quite well on the exam, even the first time around. The first Step 2 CS Examination was in June 2004. As of March 2005, there had been approximately 17,700 examinees. About half of these examinees were students from U.S. and Canadian medical schools, and about half were students or graduates of international medical schools. The overall pass rate for these U.S. and Canadian students was 96 percent and the overall pass rate for international students and graduates was 83 percent. These numbers will probably evolve as the exam matures and the examinee group grows. One of the bigger challenges of taking the exam has been the limited number of national testing sites, making expensive travel an added burden on the already financially strapped and stressed-out third-year student. Financial-aid packages now try to take this into account with additional loan monies made available, and more testing centers continue to open.

For D.O. Students It's the COMLEX Level 2

At this point in their med-school careers, D.O. students will take the next step of the COMLEX exam. Many D.O.s elect to take both the USMLE and COMLEX series in order to keep their options open. The tests are very similar and cover essentially the same scope of information. If you're taking both, by all means schedule them close together so that you have to make the study push only once. For more information on the COMLEX exam, check out the National Board of Osteopathic Medical Examiners Web site at www.nbome.org/examinations.htm.

CHAPTER 20

Elective Rotations

An investment in knowledge always pays the best interest.
—BENJAMIN FRANKLIN

ONE OF THE most astounding things about medical training is that after you achieve a foundation of knowledge, the world is literally your oyster. You are not merely encouraged but *required* to try on a wide range of fields and determine which one suits you best. Once you've completed your core rotations, you will realize how astoundingly broad the field of medicine is, and being forced to choose a single field for a career becomes both a blessing and a curse. The remainder of your third and fourth years will be dedicated to doing this through elective rotations in various fields and to building your application for residency.

Your med-school course catalog will provide an exhaustive list of available electives. There is no magic formula for which electives to choose, but the time has come to start homing in on a career choice. Be aggressive about gaining experiences in your fields of interest so that you can narrow your choices, finalize your decision, and begin to develop your residency application (see the next chapter). Talk to upperclassmen who are going into these fields and discuss with them the best elective options and best sequence of rotations. Ask them about what other fields they were considering and how they made their choices.

You need to make sure you fulfill all your curricular requirements and address any experiential requirements for your residency application, but beyond that you should have some fun and see where this senior medical student thing can take you.

You may wish to do electives in related fields to gain additional exposure that will be useful when you start your internship (e.g., radiology or infectious disease). You may also want to seek out some unique experiences you'll never get a chance to try again. Ever wonder what radiation oncology is all about? Curious about forensic pathology and the medical examiner's world? How about the numerous international electives that will provide wide-ranging experience in countries all across the world? Since some of these opportunities occur outside the confines of the U.S. medico-legal system, these rotations can give you tremendous latitude and authority as a student.

Another popular elective is the research month. If you've encountered someone along the way who is doing active research that you're interested in, see if you can set up a month to learn some hands-on clinical-research skills. Try to make sure that you define an achievable scope so that you come away with a definitive product you can use for your applications and resume (such as authorship on a paper or presentation, and so on).

The sky is truly the limit here, and most schools will give their graduating seniors considerable latitude in defining their own electives, so while you're homing in on a final selection think creatively and have fun!

PART FIVE

Applying for Residency and Surviving the Match

CHAPTER 21

Thinking About Residency

A ship in the harbor is safe, but that is not what ships were built for.
—DONALD KENDALL

THE FOURTH YEAR sneaks up on most students. You're so deeply embroiled in moving from one intense rotation to another that the time just seems to slip by. Before you know it, your third year is drawing to a close and it's time to start contemplating the road ahead again. It's time for more soul-searching to determine your specialty of choice, time to dust off your promotional skills for another round of apps, interviews, and choices.

For a minority of you, the selection of a specialty may prove an easy choice. You either remain dedicated to the direction you arrived with, or you have discovered the field along the way about which you are now utterly passionate.

More power to you if your choice is that clear.

The reality for most, however, is that there are a number of fields that seem both attractive and a good fit. This chapter will help you work through that decision-making process. It will also lay the foundation for a winning run at the residency of your choice.

MAKING THE CHOICE:
WHAT DO YOU WANT TO DO WITH YOUR LIFE?

It probably seems not that long ago that you made the decision to go to medical school. So how can you already be facing the choice of what *kind* of medicine to practice? And, more to the point, how can you base such an important decision on a few piddling weeks rotating on a service?

Oh, and what if you liked *every* rotation you did? How are you supposed to choose then?

"Much like going to medical school for the wrong reasons, if you go into a specialty you don't really enjoy, it will make you miserable," Chris notes. "Do not just look at the economic possibilities or the lifestyle or the prestige associated with certain specialties. If you do not absolutely love what you're doing, it is likely you will regret it later."

Just like applying to med school, there's no magic formula for making a decision about residency. Review your rotations and think back to the time you felt most inspired. A great place to start to gather information is the American Medical Association's fantastic Fellowship and Residency Electronic Interactive Database (FREIDA Online) Web site (www.ama-assn.org/ama/pub/category/2997.html). This Web site details every imaginable specialty, the nature of the field, the lifestyle, the compensation, and every accredited residency in the United States where it is offered. As you peruse your options, you might want to consider some criteria you should use while evaluating a specialty. We'll call them the five Ls of choosing your field.

Learning opportunities

The first question you should ask yourself is "Will I remain challenged by this field years from now?" You're about to dedicate a long career to a particular field of study. It's worth making sure you are engaged by the subject matter. This doesn't mean you have to be fascinated by every aspect of the field. It should mean, however, that you find yourself almost inexplicably drawn to the subject matter.

It should also mean that when relevance to this specialty comes up on other rotations, you find yourself a little more excited, paying a little more attention, or having a little more to offer your team in the way of expertise. The signs may be subtle at first, but you should gradually awaken to a gut feeling that this subject field resonates with you.

Think carefully about this, and figure out which field has given you the strongest positive attraction.

Long-term camaraderie

Another important part of finding your specialty is finding the right fit with the people drawn to that specialty. You'll be spending many years and many late nights with these folks, so finding a group that you seem to naturally connect with will make your life easier and more enjoyable. Even more than that, sensing that you fit well with the predominant culture of the specialty will mean your work ethic and attitudes will be more closely aligned with those of your colleagues, making your chances of success and reward that much higher.

"Sometimes you just know it's not going to work out," Pete notes. "One of my funnier experiences from residency interviews came when I asked a program about abortion training in a rural town in northern California. The interviewer stated somewhat defiantly that just last week the Planned Parenthood clinic had burned down for the third time in five years. Needless to say, I withdrew my application from the program."

Lifestyle

This may be the most crucial measure in selecting your specialty, but not just because of what it says about how well you'll succeed in that field. You *must* find a field that suits your sense of balance between work and personal life. To violate this rule is to *doom* yourself to an unhappy and ultimately unsuccessful career.

There are lots of great fields in medicine, and many outstanding physicians who accomplish incredible things on a regular basis. But if your heart is set on an intense field like trauma surgery, you must be very realistic about the impact the decision will have on your life. Consider carefully how many years of training it will take and how old you will be when you graduate. Look at the attendings around you and ask yourself if you can be happy in their job. Are *they* happy in *their* job? What is their family life like? Do they have families at all? The people who are most satisfied and successful in these high-intensity fields are the ones who scrutinized the lifestyle before they joined it and recognized and accepted the choices they would have to make.

On the other hand, you also should not select a particular specialty solely because it offers an easier lifestyle or exceptional compensation. Again, you have to be careful what you wish for. If you are entering the specialty solely because of its rewards but without a real passion for the subject matter and the patients, you will ultimately be missing out on the most important reward of all—the immense satisfaction that comes from being excited to go to work every day. Worse still, you may find yourself married to the financial gains of a field you no longer have an interest in practicing. This is a disservice to your patients, not to mention to your own life and potential.

"Don't sell yourself short in terms of personal happiness," Deb advises. "We are all so gung-ho and willing to work ourselves into the ground to prove we are dedicated. Don't underestimate the need for personal time."

Likelihood of success

Medicine is an ever-evolving field, and with each passing day the business of medicine becomes a little more complicated and a little riskier. If you're passionate about a field, you should never be dissuaded by lower salaries or fewer opportunities. On the other hand, you need to be realistic about what the prospects in your field look like both in the near-term (i.e., when you graduate) as well as twenty or thirty years down the road.

Consider the impact loan repayment will have on your monthly income and, thus, what impact it should have on your choice of career and location. Most specialties have undertaken extensive studies to determine the projected workforce needs and future job markets for their field. These studies can be a useful guide when making your decision. Try to ensure that the life you imagine building for yourself more or less matches the opportunities to succeed in the field.

"Ask a lot of questions and spend ample time within your specialty of choice," Adam suggests. "Make sure the lifestyle of the attendings and residents is in accordance with what you expect. I would advise against choosing a specialty solely on financial grounds. These things tend to change rapidly, and you risk getting bored with your choice."

Love of the particular field

This is the most nebulous of the criteria, but the list would be incomplete if it did not include a real evaluation of your sincere and reliable interest in the particular field. In choosing to go to medical school, you dedicated yourself to serving the needs of your patients. One would hope you will always bring to their bedside a passion for your work. This is a difficult thing to measure, particularly so early in your career and with such a limited exposure to the specialties you're considering. Furthermore, passion is something that grows and deepens over time as you develop experience and a broader perspective on your field. Nonetheless, if you have doubts, you'd do well to keep looking.

Even after applying these five Ls to your list of prospective specialties, you may still find yourself struggling to make a choice. Keep working at it, and keep looking for ways to eliminate some of the options. For a few people, applying to multiple specialties might be an answer. You might, for example, be tied to a specific geographic location by family. In this case, your only options in that state in your top-choice specialty may be a few extremely competitive programs. You could, therefore, apply to these programs and then broaden your list to programs in another, less competitive specialty or even a generic internship in hopes of still securing a spot within that same state.

Whatever the case, the choice must ultimately be yours, made on your own terms, and according to your own personal criteria. Do your homework, talk to mentors, talk to residents, and make your lists of pros and cons. Then, informed by all the facts, make a decision with your gut. As with most major choices in life that require a serious commitment, the decision will ultimately be at least a partial leap of faith from something you know to something you can only imagine.

In my opinion, the top five criteria that should factor into your decision are (in no particular order):
1. Lifestyle in the field (hours, call schedule, length of training, and so on)
2. Compensation
3. The needs of the community you intend to practice in

4. Academic stimulation and reward

5. Respect for and positive interactions with your peers

Look closely at the bread and butter of each specialty—as a dermatologist there are lots of rare and exotic skin conditions, but much of your day will be acne.

—Pete

DESIGNING YOUR APPLICATION SCHEDULE TO MEET YOUR GOALS

Now that you've chosen a direction, the next question is how to get there. Applications for residency are due in October of your senior year. That means that by the spring of your third year you need to be gearing up to apply. That also means you have a precious few months in the beginning of your fourth year to do some critical clinical rotations that will weigh heavily on your application.

All schools require that you complete a subinternship as a prerequisite to graduation. In your subinternship (also known as a "sub-I," or "AI" for "acting internship"), you will take on the role of an intern. You will be expected to cover more patients, to work more independently, and to bring a more experienced perspective to bear. The thrust of your evaluations of your sub-I will be an assessment of your fitness as a future intern and resident. Obviously residencies look to these evaluations for insight into what kind of resident you'll be. Therefore, it is essential that you pick a good sub-I for your field and work hard to excel in it. It is also critical to schedule this sub-I during the summer before your fourth year so that you'll have your sub-I evaluation in time for residency application season.

Many students also do an away rotation in their field of choice at residencies they are particularly interested in applying to. You definitely aren't required to do an away rotation, especially if you plan on trying to stay local for residency. However, it can offer not only serious insight into a program you're interested in but also what amounts to a month-long, in-depth interview that will have substantial bearing on your application to that residency program. Furthermore, you will develop a broader perspective on the specialty by traveling to a new site with a different faculty and a fresh perspective.

Most programs reserve a limited number of slots for medical students from other institutions, so these slots are generally hotly contested. Therefore, you should work early to identify programs you may be interested in and try to set up an away rotation early on.

When I was applying to programs I targeted my top-choice program early. I had heard it had an excellent and growing reputation, and the more research I did on the program the more intrigued I became. In April, I arranged an away rotation, filling one of the last available slots for October of that year. I had a fantastic month that confirmed everything I had heard, and I solidified my choice. I arranged to rent a spectacular seaside cottage for an end-of-season price, and I brought my wife and daughter along with me at the last moment. It worked! They too fell in love with the region, and our top choice was made.

I expressed my enthusiasm for that program both in my interview and in discussions with the residents that month. The research director ended up inviting me to stay on an extra month to help out on a last-minute research project. I was able to rearrange my school schedule and break out another elective. The second month only deepened my interest, and it offered a unique chance to hang out with residents and faculty and develop some personal friendships. Come January my decision was an easy one, and on Match Day we were thrilled to get our first choice.

—coauthor Dan

MAKING CONTACTS AND COLLECTING INFORMATION

Once you identify your specialty, you need to go into a rapid, aggressive, information-gathering mode. Scour the Internet first. Use FREIDA to find out more about the specialty in general and how it compares to other disciplines. Follow links to national organizations and societies governing that field, and read about what's current in the field on their Web sites. Finally, use the FREIDA links to go direct to residencies in that speciality. Start to narrow down a list of possible programs based on your interests, their locations, and the features they tout as their strengths.

We've mentioned at several points along the way the importance of mentorship. A good mentor can be an invaluable source of wisdom and inspiration, and a grounding influence in otherwise turbulent and confusing times. If you haven't found a mentor up to this point, do so now without fail. A mentor will be a critical element of your application process. He or she will provide critical insight on your fitness as a candidate in your specialty, advice on how to craft your application, and hopefully a strong and insightful letter of recommendation. If you already have a trusted mentor, you might consider broadening your scope within your school to include another opinion (but don't estrange your primary mentor in doing this). If you do an away rotation, you may be assigned a mentor at the outside institution who can provide this refreshingly new expert opinion. When you talk to your mentors, be sure you run your list of possible programs by them. Ask for their opinions of each program. Ask for additional programs you might not have thought about. Ask if they know anyone inside these various programs and whether they might be willing to make a call on your behalf. Try to get a sense of how competitive your preferred programs are.

Your overall list should remain quite broad at this point, but if you've started to home in on five or ten programs, start a file folder for each one and begin cataloguing your information.

Paving the Way to a Successful Match

The general schedule for your transition to fourth year should look something like this:

Third Year

March—Information Gathering
- Make your short list of possible specialties.
- Spend time talking with mentors, residents, and attendings.
- Work through your pro-and-con list.
- Do online research on residencies and the specialties.

April—Starting Out
- Arrange away rotations if desired.
- Make a contact in the department you want to specialize in and arrange a meeting. Make it clear you want to match in their specialty and are looking for mentorship and advice.

- Start asking people what kinds of activities/extra work might make your application shine in your chosen specialty—e.g., research, extra rotations, and so on.
- Sequence your schedule so that you will do your sub-I in your chosen specialty so that your remaining clerkships show strong grades.

May—Full Steam Ahead
- Try to arrange a phone call or meeting with the program director of any residencies you'll be directly targeting. Express your interest clearly but politely.
- Attempt to identify inroads to any programs you're interested in. Talk to your mentor about people he or she knows in the field who might be able to put in a good word when the time comes.
- Time to start thinking about your application. Read ahead!

You now have the pieces and parts you need to initiate a successful match at your ideal program. You've started early, weighed your options, and defined why you want to join a particular field. You've met with local faculty to gain more experience and perspective and used them to establish far-reaching contacts at other institutions. You've reached out to programs you're interested in via those contacts and politely declared your interest. You've set up an away rotation at your top-pick program.

You're ready to go.

CHAPTER 22

Applying All Over Again

Success is the progressive realization of a worthy goal or ideal.
—EARL NIGHTINGALE

THE ACTUAL APPLICATION process for residency will closely mirror your med-school application experience. By now you should be an old pro at this, so many of the tips in these chapters will be familiar.

THE SYSTEM

Applications to most allopathic residencies are standardized via the Electronic Residency Application Service (ERAS) (www.aamc.org/students/eras/start.htm), a division of the National Resident Matching Program (NRMP). More than 95 percent of residency programs use this single uniform application. The list of programs that do *not* use ERAS are listed on the ERAS Web site.

Osteopathic medical students will use a parallel match system run by the American Osteopathic Association (http://opportunities.aoa.net.org). The AOA has its own applications but runs the match through the same computer system that the NRMP uses. Osteopaths match in January, allopaths in March. Thus, it is possible for osteopathic students to participate in both matches. This discussion will focus on the allopathic match, but the osteopathic process and application is very similar.

The universal application requires you to provide a substantial amount of information, so once again it's time to start collecting your files and organizing yourself. Unlike your medical-school applications, the ERAS application will be the only application you fill out. There are *no* secondary applications in the residency process. You will work hand in hand with your medical school to register for and complete your application.

TASKS AND TIMELINES

As we noted earlier, the timeline for your residency applications should start in the spring of your third year. You should start exploring the ERAS Web site and familiarizing yourself with its tools and resources. Understand the structure of the application and its required content. Start collecting and organizing the required supporting information. By June you should begin crafting your essay and have a list of potential recommendation writers in mind.

On July 15 you will be able to use the unique log-in token supplied by your medical-school dean's office to register on the ERAS Web site and initiate your application. By early August you should have entered your personal information and your scholastic achievements and awards into ERAS. Your letter writers should be busy crafting your recommendations. Your essay should be in finalized form by mid-August, and the application should be available online by the end of August. On September 1 the residency programs you've selected will start to receive initial draft versions of your application. By November your medical school's dean's letter (explained below) will be submitted and the finalized application will be sent out to residencies. You will submit your match list in January, interview throughout the winter, and get your match results in March.

Let's break the process down into its component parts.

Crafting your application and essay

You should aim to devote the same level of painstaking attention to detail to your residency application that you did to your medical-school application. The good news is that this application is simpler, and overall the process is much more approachable. You're also wiser and more savvy about the subject matter. You've studied the spectrum of medical knowledge, you've experienced firsthand the many facets of the profession, and you've selected a particular specialty as your chosen vocation. As before, you should not only detail your academic qualifications but also strive to illustrate the path you've taken to choose your field.

There is no one ideal application. Your goal will be to demonstrate overall proficiency and to specifically highlight your unique qualities and experiences.

Once again, your personal statement will be a centerpiece of your application. Unlike your medical-school essay, your residency essay will be a focused statement of your rationale for selecting your specialty and your aspirations therein. It should demonstrate the evolution of your perspective and insight during medical school and perhaps tie in some key formative experiences. Just as with your medical-school admissions essay, the prose here must be perfect. Proof thoroughly and have several other people read your statement for content and quality.

"Remember that your personal statement is a way the reader can get to know you as a person without having met you," Deb suggests.

The dean's letter

The medical-school dean's letter is the ERAS version of your premed committee letter. The dean's letter will provide programs with a summary of your academic record and provide categorical assessment of your performance relative to your peers. This used to be a fairly subjective process, but in recent years ERAS and the various residency programs have formalized this letter to provide a uniform format and set of assessment tools.

In general, your academic record will be reviewed and your performance compared to your peers using percentages. The letter will use key phrases that correlate to certain percentages. Thus, "Curly's performance in his first two years was above average" may effectively say to programs, "Curly is in the top third of his class." Your dean's letter will also summarize your extracurricular experience and research experience. Programs will put significant weight on the dean's overall assessment of your fitness to be a future house officer (i.e., resident). Despite the efforts to standardize this letter, programs across the country will know the propensities of individual deans and will weigh their evaluations accordingly.

There's not a lot you can do to optimize your dean's letter—your record is what it is. However, you will probably have a meeting arranged with your dean sometime in the summer of your fourth year to discuss your record and the letter. Deans hold these meetings in an effort to add some personal elements to their letters and verify the accuracy of their information. As such, your dean's meeting is an opportunity for you to emphasize the elements of your application that you wish to highlight and your thoughtful and insightful reasons for pursuing your chosen field. As long as your requests are reasonable and accurately reflect your record, they will likely find their way into your letter.

Letters of recommendation

The system for letters of recommendation is slightly different in ERAS than it was for your medical-school application. If you are applying to several different types of residencies (i.e., residencies in different specialties), you will need different letters of recommendation for each specialty. Therefore, ERAS allows you to designate an unlimited number of letter writers and also allows you to select up to four letters for each program you apply to.

All letters of recommendation will be sent directly to your dean's office, which will send them to ERAS along with the dean's letter. ERAS will then send the dean's letter along with the specific letters you designate to each program. As always, plan ahead, request your letters early, and meet with each of your recommenders to help personalize your recommendation letters.

CHAPTER 23

Selecting Your Programs

The world is always willing to receive talent with open arms.
—OLIVER WENDELL HOLMES

Y OU'LL PROBABLY FIND that the trepidation you felt about selecting medical schools will be replaced with excitement when it is time to select your residency. It's a very different feeling to be on the inside looking at the next step, as opposed to being on the outside praying you'll be let in. Of course, it's still a very important choice, and one that deserves your careful consideration.

The factors influencing your choice of residency will be every bit as varied as those governing your choice of medical school. The same differentiators—location, reputation, and curriculum—will remain key factors. You will also want to consider the caliber of the faculty you'll be working with, the availability of subspecialty fellowships (if you are contemplating a subspecialty), the size of the program, the overall satisfaction of the residents in the program (termed, quaintly, "resident wellness"), the variety of the patient population, and the quality of the facilities.

Your resources for researching programs will be part digital and part personal. There is a wealth of information on the Web about every residency program in the country. Any specialty Web site will have links to the participating residencies in this field, and every residency will have its own Web page detailing its program and offering its highlights. This research makes for great late-night surfing when you're on call and waiting for lab results or waiting for a patient to arrive. In the beginning, you should just click away, exploring broadly and getting a feeling for what programs are available and what some of their basic similarities and differences are.

After a period of seemingly aimless wandering, you'll find yourself drawn back to certain Web sites again and again, holding these programs in your mind as the standard by which to judge others. These programs will merit further research for you. Start researching these more intensively and take notes on the relative strengths and weaknesses of each.

As for the personal resources, you should talk to your mentor about your program selection. Anyone who has been in the field for a period of time will have informed opinions about the various programs. As with all personal opinions, be vigilant for bias. Those who have been in academics the longest will have the broadest perspective on the field, but their opinions about specific programs may be based on facts that are no longer current. Conversely, those fresh from their training will have the most current view of the residency field and will have very up-to-date information on specific programs. Yet these same folks may hold strong opinions based on their personal experience in the program they just graduated from instead of a knowledge of the field as a whole.

APPLYING AS A COUPLE

It's not uncommon for romance to blossom in the trenches of medical school. Let's face it, you've been through an extensive vetting process just to get into school. For the last several years, you've been surrounded by several hundred fellow Type A personalities who are smart, driven, and equally passionate about health care. You've enjoyed the camaraderie that comes from surviving the trials and tribulations of med school that are simply inexplicable to the uninitiated. But with the end of school looming nearer and nearer, choices have to be made.

If you have a paramour in your med-school class, your first decision is whether to lay out your future as a couple. If you're married, this is obviously a nonissue—but if you're just seriously dating, this is going to put you to a choice. Residency is a stressful time, and not being in the same location will make maintaining a relationship virtually impossible. On the other hand, committing to move to the same place for your training is making a statement about the direction of your relationship. If the relationship later doesn't work out, you may be left in very close working proximity with each other.

Needless to say, this choice requires careful thought and open, honest discussion.

The NRMP does provide a vehicle for couples trying to match together. As you apply to programs, you can select to apply as a couple, either in the same specialty or in different specialties at the same institution. This means when you rank a program on your list, it will be coordinated with your partner's match list, and the NRMP computers will attempt to match you to these coordinated programs. This definitely adds an additional layer of complexity to an already intricate process, but many people do it successfully each year. The challenge tends to be finding programs that both people are interested in, can get interviews at, and can rank equally.

If you're applying to a program as a couple's match, be sure to alert the program to this. Within the institution, the program you apply to will coordinate their interview dates with your partner's program and will also discuss their relative rankings of your respective candidacies when it comes time to complete their list. Thus, if one of you is held in particularly high esteem by a program, the residency director may pull strings to help ensure that your partner gets ranked favorably in the other program as well.

Making Your Final List

The final list of programs to which you apply will be shaped by many of the aforementioned factors and probably by several others that you uncover along the way. The list of residency programs you apply to will obviously be broader than the list of programs you rank when it comes time to register for the match. That said, you should resist the urge to apply to every single program in your specialty in the country.

The shotgun approach is tempting, especially if you're filled with that all-too-familiar paranoia that you might not get in anywhere. In the end, though, the shotgun approach is a self-defeating strategy. First, it's a disservice to yourself. You've worked hard to get where you are, and you should have some faith in your strength as a candidate. Target programs that are realistic for you, but recognize that those programs are seeking to recruit you as well. The days of hoping for an admission should be left behind. Your goal should be finding the best possible match between your strengths and goals as a candidate and the programs you're looking at.

Second, applying to every single program in the country is a disservice to your fellow applicants and to the system as a whole. It suggests you haven't given due consideration to the field and narrowed your choices, and by applying everywhere you may be limiting someone else's chances at getting an interview at a program they love but one you may not even be interested in.

CHAPTER 24

Residency Interviews

I am not now
That which I have been.
—LORD BYRON

DUST OFF YOUR suit and polish your smile. It's time to hit the interview trail again.

After several weeks of waiting with bated breath, residency-interview offers will start to arrive. As you wait, spend some time refreshing your interview skills. Remember all that practice in talking confidently about yourself and your application? Remember developing insightful questions for each program? Your residency interviews will be very similar to your medical-school interviews. Begin your preparation by turning back to chapter 8 and reviewing the basics.

HOW THEY'RE DIFFERENT FROM ADMISSIONS INTERVIEWS

The good news is that your residency interviews will be much less stressful than your medical-school-admissions interviews were. You're much more knowledgeable now, and you've already gained some practical experience in the field you want to pursue. If you've been offered an interview, you know that you've passed the threshold academic criteria for the program.

Good programs will make you feel immediately welcomed. There will typically be a presentation and tour that give the program a chance to strut its stuff and highlight its strengths. The interview segment will follow, which truthfully is more a series of conversations than an inquisition. The fundamental goal here for both sides is to determine fit. Unlike your life in medical school, you'll be working many, many hours with the same relatively small group of people, so it becomes imperative for both sides that personalities mesh and work ethic aligns. In the small confines of a residency program, a single problem resident can be a disaster.

INTERVIEW TACTICS

Interviewing is very much a two-way street. You project a certain persona, and in turn you take away an impression of the interviewer and the program as a whole. When you sit down with a residency interviewer, you want to make certain that you leave a strong overall impression and convey one or two key things you want them to remember as they go back to discuss that day's candidates.

Projecting an overall image has a lot to do with your body language, your tone, and the flow of the conversation. Obviously you want to be open, friendly, and confident without being cocky. Try also to be relaxed without being a slouch. Your enthusiasm for the specialty and program must shine through. In almost any interview, you will be given some sort of open-ended question to highlight your record or your perspective. Have in mind two or three key points that you want to make sure the interviewer walks away with. Be clear and concise. At this point you should have a growing perspective on the specialty, so make it clear you have some specific goals for your future in the field.

"Be yourself in the interview," Kate advises. "The residency knows how you look on paper. Now they want to find out how you are in person—can you interact well, are you poised, can you communicate? Are you a fit for their program? What else do you enjoy besides medicine? Can you hold a conversation? Sounds simple, but it's probably the most important aspect of your application. So be you. Be honest. Avoid prescripted answers."

How to Evaluate Programs

The impression you take away from a program will be the result of your interviews and experiences. You should cover some key questions as you evaluate each program on your list in order to develop better this impression and to compare and contrast individual programs. First, do the residents in the program seem happy? Have many left the program, and if so why? How stable is the faculty roster? Has the program achieved accreditation by the Accreditation Council for Graduate Medical Education (ACGME, at www.acgme.org), meaning that it is an approved residency program? If not, where did it fail, and what is being done to remedy the situation? Even if it achieved accreditation, were there any concerns or areas of improvement noted at the last review? What is the patient population like, and what is the resident workload like? Will you see enough volume and diversity to satisfy your training requirements? Will you see too much volume to allow any time for teaching? What are the facilities like? What is the program's policy on moonlighting? Where have the program's graduates gotten jobs or fellowships?

These are just a few of the questions you might want to ask. You'll add to this list as you become a more experienced interviewer and gain more perspective on the ubiquitous and the unique in each program you review.

"Prepare good questions to ask, as the interview day is really structured to inform you about a program," Adam suggests. "Do not ask inane questions just to appear interested. We had a student ask several different residents how much they paid for parking. Who cares? This did not make the best impression. It's like asking how many books are in the library."

Scheduling Your Interviews

Scheduling your interviews will prove a challenge, just as it was in the medical-school process. It seems like no matter how much you try to orchestrate your interviews, you'll still be crisscrossing the country trying to fit them all in efficiently. This is a time-consuming and costly process. Most schools offer additional financial-aid loans to senior students to help cover the costs of travel for interviews.

The farther you get down the interview trail, the more informed a consumer you will become. Toward the end of your interview sequence, you may feel you want to curtail your remaining list somewhat in light of what you've already seen. Providing you've covered a good range of options already, including some top choices and some safer choices, this may be a reasonable thing to do. As always, you should alert a program as soon as you're sure you're going to decline their offer to interview so that others can take your spot. If you've been wait-listed for an interview anywhere, make sure you check in with the program frequently and reassert your interest. Don't pester and don't be overbearing, but do remain active and politely enthusiastic. By the end of the interview season, many candidates start canceling interviews, and programs begin calling people from their interview wait list. If you're patient and persistent, chances are good you'll get your interview.

Just as it was with medical-school interviews, your postinterview follow-up letter is key to your overall strategy. Immediately after spending the day at a program, you should write a thank-you note to the program director and to any interviewers with whom you felt you made a good personal connection. The note should be brief, succinct, friendly, and professional. Where possible, customize each note to reflect some specifics from your experience or from your conversation with that person.

As the season progresses you will start to get a feel for which programs you're especially interested in. When communicating with your top-choice programs, you must strike that delicate balance between leaving a lasting impression and making your name familiar to the residents and faculty, without being overbearing or pushy. You may want to contact some residents with specific follow-up questions. Another excellent technique can be scheduling a "second look" visit. This is an opportunity for you to visit the program on a noninterview day, to spend some more time clinically with the residents, and to chat some more with the program director and faculty. This will help cement you in their minds, and may offer you a deeper insight into the program, confirming or dispelling your initial interest.

Another key to keeping your application fresh in the program director's mind is to continually update your file. Anytime you receive awards or accolades, anytime you get an article published or have some particularly unique experience, update your ERAS file and

CHAPTER 25

The Match

The die is cast!
—SUETONIUS

WITH INTERVIEWS NOW under your belt, it's time to put together your match list. This is the sequential ranking of programs you applied to and interviewed at. Once you assemble this list, the NRMP will combine your list with each program's corresponding list to match you to the highest-ranked program on your list that offered you a spot. This list, therefore, is critically important. Follow these few simple rules to make creating your list a snap and ensure you match at the best place you can.

MAKING YOUR LIST

The fundamental rule to making your list is: be honest. It's tempting to try to game the system, hedging on the algorithm by ranking programs you're especially excited about slightly further down your list on the misguided notion that you probably won't get your first choice but are likely to get your second, third, or fourth choices. Don't play games with the process—it just isn't worth doing.

The simple way to construct the ideal rank list is to sit down with the list of places you interviewed and organize them according to where you want to go. Look over the list, reflect on why you applied to each program and how your experiences there did or did not confirm your interest. Write out a list of pros and cons for each program, if that helps. Talk it through with a friend, a family member, a trusted classmate, or your mentor. Review the criteria for selecting a program discussed in the previous chapter and reaffirm what the most important features of your ideal program are—these may have changed now that you've interviewed and have a much broader perspective on residencies and the specialty.

Now make your list. Just like that, write it all down, number one to however many programs you have, and then put your list aside and walk away for a day or two.

After a couple of days, pick a quiet hour and sit down with the list one more time. Glance down at your top three choices and gauge your visceral response to these programs.

Do you get a tingle of excitement at the idea of going to these programs?

Now look down at the next seven programs. Still kinda tingly? Still some pretty cool places?

Perfect.

Now look over the entire list and ask yourself this *critical* question: is there *any program* on that list that you would *not* be excited to go to if you matched? If there is, drop that program from your list. Remember that the match is a binding contract, and you could theoretically end up at *any* program on your list. Life is too short to spend a residency somewhere you don't want to be. Strike all programs about which you have uncertainties from your list before you submit it.

Assuming that you've carefully considered your options, surveyed the field, interviewed and discussed the various programs, and crafted your rank list, go to the ERAS Web site (www.aamc.org/students/eras/start.htm), type in your list, check it for accuracy, and hit "Submit."

You're done.

Walk away with a grin and the knowledge that you're going to end up somewhere you're excited to go. Spend the next few weeks focusing on your rotations and enjoying your senior year. Let go of the stress and strain of the match—it will take care of itself and there's nothing more you can do about it.

MATCH NUMBERS AND "THE SCRAMBLE"

Though you can't do anything about it, you're not technically out of the woods completely once your rank list is submitted. As the

NRMP cranks through everyone's rank lists, it does run into scenarios where there is no achievable match for a candidate or where it is unable to fill all the positions in a given program. In these cases the process reverts to good old-fashioned human networking.

Welcome to "The Scramble."

Match Day is typically mid-March, usually around the eighteenth of the month. Several days prior to this, NRMP will alert you whether or not you matched. It won't tell you where you matched, just whether or not you did. If you failed to match, you will automatically be eligible for The Scramble.

In this minimatch process, all of the available candidates ("free agents," if you will) are posted on a Web site along with all the unfilled programs. At an appointed hour, applicants across the country can start calling those unfilled programs. Materials are then faxed frantically, and rapid interviews occur over the phone.

Ideally, a good fit is found between an unfulfilled program and a free agent candidate, and both parties win.

Every fourth-year medical student lives in fear of The Scramble. There's something about medical students that seems to make them *seek* opportunities to be paranoid and pessimistic. The reality, thankfully, is in your favor.

According to the AAMC, there were 14,719 active applicants from U.S. medical schools enrolled in the 2005 allopathic match. Of these, 93.7 percent matched successfully. Thus only 6.3 percent, or 921 students, were forced into The Scramble. Most of these students did not match primarily because of problems with their match lists—either their list didn't get submitted on time, if at all (a particularly embarrassing situation to be avoided at all cost), they had an extremely limited rank list, or they applied only to extraordinarily competitive programs in a competitive field without any fall-back choices.

If you follow the advice detailed above, you will avoid most, if not all, of these scenarios.

The numbers are less favorable for non-U.S. medical-school graduates. For Canadian students in the U.S. match, the scramble rate was 27.1 percent; for osteopaths, 31.4 percent; and for foreign graduates, 45.3 percent. If you are applying from one of these groups, it is critical that you play your cards carefully and make a strong impression at your top-choice programs. Your best bet will be figuring out a way to make yourself someone the program can't imagine living without.

If for whatever reason you find yourself in The Scramble, fear not. Out of chaos can come surprising opportunity. Every year, strong and reputable programs fail to fill completely. There are always highly desirable positions available through The Scramble, and with a little effort and quick action you may be surprised to find yourself matched to a program you didn't even think you had a shot at. Your dean or faculty advisor should be at your side as The Scramble opens to assist you through the process and to help you make your choices. These faculty members have helped scores of others before you through The Scramble, so trust their advice.

In the end, although The Scramble may feel scary, you might just be surprised how well it all works out.

MATCH DAY

At long last, the day of reckoning is upon you. All those years, all those hours of studying are about to culminate in your acceptance to a residency, and your ticket to specialty training and your career in medicine. Most schools have a Match Day ceremony in which you will gather in a large hall with your classmates and open your acceptance letters. This is a dramatic and festive occasion. On the one hand, you are sad to be leaving your classmates and your medical-school experiences behind. On the other hand . . . *hallelujah!!!* You're free! You survived! The last piece of this medical-career puzzle has fallen into place.

CHAPTER 26

Finishing Up

There will come a time when you believe everything is finished.
That will be the beginning.
—LOUIS L'AMOUR

THE LAST FEW weeks of school will go by all too quickly. Your primary focus will, appropriately, be on making the transition to your new life post–medical school. With all of your core requirements completed, you can focus on having fun and relaxing.

ELECTIVE TIME: HAVE FUN, TRY SOMETHING DIFFERENT

Obviously if you have remaining required rotations that must be completed prior to graduation, focus on getting those done immediately. If you have elective time to fill, you might want to consider drumming up some unique experiences you might not get another opportunity to pursue. Travel and international electives are a popular way to round out your medical-school experience and provide very different perspective on health care as a whole. You may be able to arrange a wilderness-medicine elective, or even a liberal-arts elective to focus on a creative endeavor related to medicine.

Deans are typically fairly liberal with what they will allow in these last few months, providing you can demonstrate some medical relevance. Many schools offer preinternship didactic reviews like "Pharmacology for Interns" or "Effective Laboratory Testing." These can be helpful reviews, and typically have a very light class schedule that gives you plenty of free time. Finally, you should consider pursuing any last-minute interests or curiosities before you leave the medical-school nest altogether. In general you will want to avoid intensely time-consuming or exhausting electives at this point. Do you *really* need another month of critical care now? You'll have plenty of that in a few months' time when internship starts.

VACATION!

Most people have a fair amount of vacation stored up toward the end of their senior year. Take it! Enjoy the opportunity to spend longer periods of free time with friends, family, and loved ones. Travel if you can. Get outside. Get back in shape. Get yourself centered and healthy in body and mind.

It will all start again soon enough!

CERTIFICATIONS

Many schools offer some transitional certification classes that can save you time once you get to residency. All residents are required to be certified in Advanced Cardiac Life Support (ACLS) and/or Pediatric Advanced Life Support (PALS). Many services may also require Advanced Trauma Life Support (ATLS). There will be mechanisms in place in your residency to acquire all the certifications you need when you start. Nonetheless, if you can check these classes off your list before you leave medical school it may save you some time when you start your internship. You can contact the coordinator or program director at your new residency for information on what certifications you'll be required to have.

FINANCIAL AID CONSIDERATIONS

Finally, before you leave medical school you will be required to have an exit interview with your financial-aid advisor. This will be an opportunity to review your total loan package, the repayment requirements, and your options for deferment or forbearance. Federal law requires a financial-aid advisor to have this meeting with you to ensure that you are aware of your obligations regarding your loans.

Spend some time prior to this meeting organizing your files and bringing yourself up-to-date on your financial-aid package. If you have additional credit card or other outstanding debt, gather these records and try to formulate a plan for repaying or managing this debt as well.

When you meet with your financial-aid advisor, review your complete financial picture and discuss how your loans fit into this. Find out if there are any unique loans in your package that mature at different times or have unusual repayment requirements. It is absolutely critical that you be organized and on top of your loans prior to leaving medical school. The next chapter will delve more deeply into the key loan-management tasks you should accomplish before starting work. Once you start your internship, you want these things to be on autopilot so you don't have to spend your precious free time stressing about the details.

PART SIX

The Transition to
Residency and
Life as a Physician

CHAPTER 27

Making the Leap

The trouble with getting a life is making the payments.
—UNKNOWN

GRADUATION IS FAST becoming a hazy memory, and the celebratory headache is finally starting to fade. You now proudly list M.D. or D.O. after your name. Since med schools typically graduate in mid-to-late May but your residency won't start until the last week of June, you find yourself staring at a few precious weeks to pack up shop and make a new life for yourself as an intern. Just like the transition to medical school, take advantage of this small interlude and organize yourself in preparation for the onslaught—you'll thank yourself later.

SETTING UP SHOP

Start with the basics—make yourself a home and headquarters. If you're staying in the same town or area, you may not need to move at all. Then again, new digs, with or without roommates, may be a refreshing change. Residents don't make much, but you may find you can afford a step up in housing on your new salary.

If you're moving to a new area, it'll be worth rereading the sections of this book on finding a home in a new area. The same considerations will apply. The primary principles for all that you do should again be *safety, convenience,* and *simplicity.* Your schedule will be so hectic and your fatigue often so great that having a long commute or complicated living situation is to be avoided at all costs.

Organizing Your Life

Get your new life up and running as quickly as possible. Find an apartment or house near the hospital that is simple, safe, and low-maintenance. Get your bank account set up and activate direct deposit for your paycheck. Establish online banking so you can pay your bills at odd hours and on Sundays; or, better still, set up automatic payments for as many bills as possible so you don't even have to worry about them. Be sure to make allowances in your budget for time off, time away, and time to work out and remain in shape.

Now more than ever, balance is key.

Managing Your Loans

Your financial-aid exit interview should have made clear that qualifying for and accumulating debt is easy—but repayment is a bitch. Thankfully there are ways you can put off this problem until you are out of training and have a more substantial income.

As noted in chapter 11, your loan package will come in two major forms—subsidized and unsubsidized loans. None of your loans will require repayment prior to graduation, but your unsubsidized loans *do* begin to accrue interest. You've already watched these loan balances balloon with each passing statement.

Now is the time to be proactive in managing this debt.

If you're interested in any of the repayment options such as the National Health Service Corps or the military, you can still enroll to immediately reduce or even eliminate your debt burden. But even if these options aren't for you, read on as we discuss strategies for managing your loans.

The first step, as always, is to get everything in order. Hopefully your loan files are still well organized from your discussions with your financial-aid advisor at your exit interview. If you haven't already, make yourself a spreadsheet of all the loans in your financial-aid package, their total amount, and the date they go into active repayment. Make sure all the lenders have a current address for you once you get established. The last thing you want is creditors hunting you down because a lender can't find you and puts you in default on a loan you didn't know was due.

If you're like most students, the bulk of your package will be federal loans, with a few Perkins or private loans added in. You may want to scrutinize these nonfederal loans first. If they're for smaller dollar amounts and you can afford to do it, you may want to consider paying them off at this point. This will simplify your mix of loans and make the next steps, consolidation and repayment, easier.

Most federal loans go into repayment six months after you cease being a full-time student. Unfortunately, your graduate training in internship and residency does *not* qualify you as a student. Thus, you will be expected to start making payments on your student loans halfway through your internship. For most, this is not a tenable position, as a resident's already small salary won't stretch far to cover a hefty loan payment. That's the bad news. The good news is there are key ways you can both reduce and defer these payments.

Your first and most critical action should be to consolidate the many loans in your package into a single jumbo loan. This will allow you to do three things: first, you will have to make only a single loan payment each month to the consolidator, which simplifies your paperwork and accounting; second, the consolidated loan will be locked in at a single interest rate, allowing you to more accurately budget and plan; and finally, and most important, because the consolidated lender will have a much larger loan they will offer you a much more favorable rate. This will save you *tens of thousands of dollars* over the life of the loan.

Do not fail to take this critical step.

There are many ways to consolidate your loan, and your mailbox will literally be inundated with offers. The federal government has its own consolidation program through the Direct Loans Servicing Agency (www.dlservicer.ed.gov) for consolidation of federal loans. If you have private loans and equity lines, you will need to consolidate these through a private lender. Several large private lending institutions like Sallie Mae and Washington Mutual also offer private consolidation packages. While their rates and terms are not as good as the federal consolidation service, they are still considerably better than your individual unconsolidated loans would be. In the end, you should shop around and identify the best offer with the lowest fixed rate—but be on the lookout for hidden consolidation fees and costs that might make an amazing offer too good to be true. Also note that the federal consolidation program has options that allow you to defer your loan payment further (this is discussed below). Some private lenders offer this, but some don't, so investigate thoroughly before you commit.

Now that you've shed the tiny loans and consolidated the remainder into one low-interest megaloan, you're ready to worry about the fact that you *still* can't figure out how you'll afford even the reduced monthly payments.

You have some options here as well.

There are two ways to avoid immediate repayment on federal loans. The first, and certainly the best financial option, will be to apply for economic hardship deferment. If you have prior student loans (i.e., from your undergraduate days) and you make below a set salary, you may qualify to defer payment on any of your loans *interest free*.

Wow.

You will have to reapply for economic hardship deferment every year to ensure that you qualify for the program.

If you don't have prior student loans or otherwise don't qualify for economic hardship, you may instead elect to go into forbearance. Forbearance requires you to affirm to the government that you remain financially incapable of repaying your loans right now, and to pledge to assume payments as soon as you can. Your loans will continue to accrue interest, and, in fact, you'll continue to get bills in the mail for your payments. But as long as you're in forbearance, you won't be required to repay a cent.

At the end of the forbearance period, you will resume payments on the full amount, including the interest you've accrued. This is a decidedly less ideal solution, but it at least buys you the time to get your training done and a real salary in place.

Finally, and as always, *stay* organized. Life's about to get hectic again, so keep your files in order and stay on top of your loan responsibilities. These are big numbers with serious consequences, so make it a priority to stay on top of deadlines and keep yourself in the clear. You'll rest easier knowing your loans are under control.

CHAPTER 28

Starting Out Strong in Residency

There is a certain relief in change, even though it be from bad to worse!
As I have often found in traveling in a stagecoach, that it is often a comfort
to shift one's position, and be bruised in a new place.
—WASHINGTON IRVING

BY NOW YOU'VE been through this transition thing a number of times. You know it feels terrifying initially, but then you get your feet under you and you begin to realize you really can handle Orgo, or Anatomy, or the boards, or your first day on the wards, or . . . your first day of internship. There is no doubt that you are making a major transition from medical school to residency, but if you take it one step at a time everything will fall into place.

ORIENTATION

Your first day will be July 1. About a week or so prior to this, however, you will probably have orientation activities arranged by your new program. Most of these activities will be administrative tasks like getting your ID and new white coats, but there will be some social events with the other residents and your new classmates thrown in. You'll probably also have some basic didactics to help you get on your feet. The didactics will focus on common conditions you will encounter and common problems that may arise on call and on the wards. The week will be a general blur, filled with new people, new places, and too much information to handle. Don't worry. Absorb what you can and assume you'll pick up the rest along the way.

YOUR FIRST DAY ON THE WARDS

Getting used to a new hospital is never easy. Then again, you've become a professional at reinventing yourself with every new rotation you encountered. Jumping into a new team with a new set of responsibilities will feel surprisingly familiar by this point. Plus, everyone around you will be going through exactly the same thing. Take your time, be honest about what you don't know or don't feel comfortable doing, and things will fall into place.

While the hospital environment will feel familiar, you may be struck by the degree to which your workload has changed. Your senior residents will quickly start piling on the patients, and before you know it, you'll have a juggling act going. The first time your pager goes off, you'll pretty much jump out of your skin. You'll nervously dial the number and have to suppress the urge to say you're a medical student returning a page. Chances are it will be some prosaic question that the nurse pretty much could have answered on his or her own. Nonetheless, you'll jump to the task with pride, eager to make a strong first impression.

Then it will go off again.

And again.

Pretty soon you'll start wondering how you're going to get anything done with that thing attached to your hip. Just as you're admitting your fourth patient of the day, you'll get paged from the floor that someone's blood pressure is 70 and they're not breathing too well.

Uh-oh. Then you'll get paged by your resident telling you there's another admission coming in twenty minutes.

Then your attending will call to ask if you've finished the first admission and whether or not you're ready to discuss the case.

And somewhere around then, you'll feel a bead of perspiration run down your forehead and suddenly find it difficult to swallow. Don't worry. You'll get comfortable, get into the rhythm of your service, and get infinitely more efficient.

YOUR FIRST CALL NIGHT

The looming responsibility of call will first dawn on you at evening sign-out. Your team will gather and you'll step through the patient list for the entire service, listening to the bullet-item highlights on each patient and anything that needs to be done overnight. "Mr. Harmon is recovering from a GI bleed. Keep his pressures below 140 systolic and check a hematocrit that has been ordered for midnight. Transfuse for anything less than 20 percent."

"Uh, okay," you say. "How do I check a timed lab? And how do I order a blood transfusion?"

In the meantime, you're already at the next patient and the resident is expanding your already burgeoning to-do list. Just keep scribbling away and make yourself check boxes for each task you need to complete. You've got the rest of the night to track down results and keep everyone alive.

That first night will be a long and sleepless one. You'll probably get several admissions that you'll handle with your team, all the while being paged continuously from the floor. Your history and physical notes will be long and a little shaky. When you do finally lay your head down in the call room, your pager will go off.

A basic rule of call nights is: when in doubt, go see the patient in person. Answer the question after you've had a chance to look through the chart and get some perspective on the case. Let yourself build some experience before being cavalier about answering questions and ordering meds on patients you know relatively little about. If you have doubts or concerns, don't feel awkward about calling your senior resident or attending. They're expecting this. Better by far to speak up and ask a stupid question than to be proven a fool when you make a silent guess and put a patient in jeopardy.

Morning will come with agonizing slowness. As your team files in for morning sign-out, you'll again step through your list, reporting on the events of the night for each patient.

Now you get to start a regular day and go right into prerounds, get your notes written, and then slow-walk rounds with the team. As fatigue overcomes you, you'll find yourself leaning against doorways while you listen to other presentations, drifting into half sleep, only to be jarred awake periodically by a sudden pimping question.

At long last, rounds will end and you'll sign out your patients to a fellow team member and get to go home. This will usually be around noon. When you get home, unplug your phone, turn off your pager, and crash into your own, peaceful, undisturbed bed for some much-needed and much-deserved rest.

Congrats! You survived your first call night.

Now get some sleep so you can do it all again tomorrow.

UNDERSTANDING ACADEMICS IN RESIDENCY

Unfortunately your dreams of putting the books up on the shelf once and for all are just that—fantasies. Studying will be a persistent activity throughout your residency. True, it will come in different forms, but regular reading and didactic learning will be fundamental to your overall education in residency. While you may be employed by the hospital as a clinician, you're still very much a student of medicine. You should be reading about the cases that you encounter, on a daily basis if possible.

Your lectures in residency will come in the form of weekly didactic conferences. Some programs have one or two hours a day; others block the lectures into a single day a week. The conferences will be led mostly by faculty members, and each hour will typically cover a different topic germane to your field of study. Some will be given by fellow residents, and, indeed, as you progress in your training you will be asked to prepare and deliver more and more of these. These are the same conferences you sat through as a medical student while on various rotations—only now, you'll be a resident sharing the hot seat for pimping questions. At least once a month you'll probably have some sort of "Morbidity and Mortality" conference in which critical cases are dissected and the errors or opportunities for improvement discussed candidly. These can be painful, especially when a case you were involved with turned out badly, but this is also some of the most poignant learning you will ever do.

We all learn through our mistakes—and nowhere is this more humbling than in medicine.

Finally, you'll probably meet monthly at a restaurant as a resident group for a "Journal Club." You'll have a few beers and discuss some articles from the literature.

You will also have an annual in-service exam that is meant to be a precursor to the specialty board exam you'll take after you graduate from residency. To prepare for the in-service, and to get you on track for your boards, you should find a good board review book for your specialty and systematically work your way through it. It will seem painful to continue the drudgery of textbook reading, but incremental efforts throughout your years as a resident will pay big dividends in the end. Furthermore, staying abreast of your field will be a lifelong pursuit, so working now to instill good reading habits will serve you and your patients for years to come.

Most programs will impose one final requirement on their residents—an academic project. This is typically some form of research project and presentation to be completed during their training. The definitions for this project are usually fairly broad and are meant to include everything from original clinical research to case reports to quality assessment studies. You'll probably be required to prepare a report or presentation on the project. Ideally you'll be able to present your project at a national meeting. At first the project will seem like a huge undertaking. But take a minute and talk to the more senior residents about what they've done. Talk to your faculty members about their research interests and ongoing projects. Chances are that before you know it you will find an idea blossoming in your head. Curiosity is a healthy attribute in a physician, and this is a great opportunity to explore your horizons a little.

Speaking of horizons, it is worth reminding yourself on a daily basis that you are now embarking on a career. You've landed in your specialty, and as you progress through your residency you are laying the foundation for years to come. Be diligent, be inquisitive, and strive to hone your skills and knowledge. You are in an incredibly rich academic environment with a group of highly skilled and dedicated faculty whose sole purpose is to teach you, often one-on-one at the bedside. Learn from these people. Get to know them. Ask them about their lives and their careers. Explore the subtleties of your specialty and ask what's available from the profession. You'll probably find there are subspecialties, offshoots, and opportunities you never knew existed. Contemplate whether you want to join the academic ranks and continue a career of research and teaching or whether you want to pursue community medicine and its very real rewards.

THE BALANCING POINT

Month will follow month, and before you know it you'll be halfway through your intern year. What once seemed impossible to contemplate has now become the mundane. No longer a stranger to day-in-day-out patient care and now disturbingly attuned to sleep deprivation and life in a call room, you may ask yourself, "When did I become an inmate in this crazy game?"

The answer, as you know, lies in the murky past, some five or six years ago, when you picked up this book and thought, "Hmmm . . . maybe medicine?"

But take heart! Life will get better. Many would say the midpoint of your intern year is an absolute nadir in life. This year, your life has been led way out on a limb of extreme work and fatigue. You've found yourself running in the same loop from home to work to home, seemingly without pause. It's *normal* to feel trapped. All this rhetoric about maintaining balance is great, but some days just maintaining a modicum of sanity will be the goal. You must weather the storm by whatever means you can. Talk to your peers and you will probably begin to realize you are not alone in these feelings. Recognize the progress you are making and just keep putting one foot in front of the other. Try as best you can to stick to the plan you set out with at the beginning of the year, including the goals for exercise, for time with friends, and for time to yourself.

If you find yourself in a downward spiral or making choices you know in your heart are not wise, seek help immediately. Depression, substance abuse, and other self-destructive behaviors are not uncommon among interns. Just as in medical school, there are people and programs available in your residency, in your hospital, and in your community to help you overcome these hurdles and get back to that track you set yourself on originally. Have the courage to admit you need help and address any issues as soon as you can, before they become unmanageable or derailing.

THE USMLE STEP 3 EXAM

The final test is upon you.

In order to qualify for the USMLE Step 3 Exam you must have completed one year of postgraduate training (i.e., an internship). Most people take the Step 3 Exam in the summer after their intern year, when all the basics are still fresh in their heads. At this point, you're probably not sure whether to cry or leap for joy knowing that the last of these monsters is finally here. The good news is that you've already completed 90 percent of your preparation for this test before you even crack a review book. The Step 3 Exam attempts to focus on your ability to actually manage patient care. Just by spending the last three years of your life in the trenches, you've developed an impressive arsenal of real-world clinical knowledge that cannot be gleaned from books. You'll bring this new skill set to bear on the Step 3 Exam.

According to the USMLE, the goal of the Step 3 Exam is to "determine if a physician possesses and can apply the medical knowledge and understanding of clinical science considered essential for the unsupervised practice of medicine, with emphasis on patient management in ambulatory-care settings." Essentially they've already taken great pains to make you prove you're smart and can memorize a tremendous volume of relatively useless information, so now, after all this time and all the money you've paid for these exams, they're *finally* going to test what you do as a physician.

It's about time.

Unfortunately they're primarily going to test what you do if you're a primary-care physician, which does cover many fundamentals of clinical medicine but may or may not apply well to your particular specialty. If you have your heart set on being a urologist, you may need to spend some time reviewing and rehearsing the management of things like hypertension, diabetes, and other common illnesses in preparation for the exam.

The exam itself is also a little different from the prior USMLE exams. The test falls over two eight-hour days. The first day will be spent fending off 336 multiple-choice questions broken into seven sections. These will be relatively typical USMLE multiple-choice questions. The second day will start with another 144 multiple-choice questions in four blocks over the first three hours. After these, you will change gears and go through a series of computer case simulations on the USMLE's Primum simulation software. You will work through about nine cases over four hours.

The Primum software allows you to work through a patient encounter that may span as long as several weeks. Essentially you will be given the chief complaint, vital signs, and pertinent history in a typical appearing triage note. You will then interview and examine the patient by selecting from a list of possible questions and exams. The results of your investigations will be made available in real time. If you order blood work on a patient and you're working in your "office," you won't get the results until the next day. Thankfully the nice folks at USMLE recognized that overnighting at the test center might be awkward, so they included a button that allows you to speed up time. Thus you will see a new patient, order a test, make a provisional diagnosis, and move forward in time as you see fit until you have test results, or you wish to reexamine the patient, or the patient's condition changes. Some cases will occur in your "office," some will occur in the "hospital." You may elect to admit someone from your office to the hospital, in which case you will follow them and be their physician during their inpatient stay.

The software generally uses free-text entry for orders and questions, allowing you considerable freedom in working with the patient. The software is trying to make sure you achieve certain milestones in the case at appropriate times. Once you've completed the milestones the case will conclude. If you fail to complete the milestones in the allotted time, the case will still close and you will move on to the next patient.

Studying for the Step 3 Exam is, obviously, very different from studying for the other Step Exams. By and large, the multiple-choice questions cover fundamental clinical knowledge that you'll probably be familiar with. You should get a good general Step 3 reference book to help you review the essential concepts and make sure you bone up on some of the facts that might be growing a little hazy. Again, this is especially true if your internship has been in a non-primary-care field where you have not been dealing with these basic problems day in and day out.

The best way to study for the case simulation portion of the test is to spend time getting comfortable with the Primum software. The USMLE allows you to download the software and a series of example cases. Spend time working through these and getting very used to the controls and quirks of the program. The software is by no means perfect, and in many cases you'll get frustrated by its lack of realism, but in the end you'll probably find that it's a bit like playing a glorified video game.

Pass rates for the Step 3 Exam are the highest of any USMLE exam. More than 95 percent of residents from U.S. and Canadian schools passed on their first attempt. It's worth some studying so you don't get surprised by the content or format of the test, but don't make yourself crazy over this one. All of the hard work you've been doing over the last five years will pay dividends here.

THE FUTURE

Take a moment to appreciate what you've done.

Internship has drawn to a close. The last USMLE Step Exam is behind you. As a clinician, you've grown from a hesitant, halting med student to develop your own relaxed and effective style with patients. As a resident, you've watched a cadre of new fourth-year medical students parade through your program, praying for a spot like yours come Match Day. Now you're preparing to make the jump to second year and your first chance to take on a more pivotal role in the care team.

The fun is about to begin.

Remember when you first got to medical school and you were awestruck by how far the horizon seemed to stretch? You could go in any one of a million directions, and all around you were people dedicated to showing you the way. Since that time, you've locked in on some specific niches that appealed to your strengths and interests. You're well on the path to becoming an expert in your arena. But the amazing thing you're probably also discovering is that the horizon remains almost as limitless.

Yes, you've narrowed your focus and you may now have responsibilities and life choices that constrain your options, but no matter where you stand there is an incredibly broad array of options for someone with your skills. You may decide to stay in clinical medicine or make a foray into research. You may decide to teach and enter an academic career. You may decide to get involved in business and technology, or you may decide to focus on medical relief and international medicine. Whatever your choice, and whatever your interests, there is almost certainly a way to pursue it and a place where your skills are in need.

It has been a long and hard road to travel. You deserve credit and respect for your dedication and perseverance. Your just reward is to be counted among the lucky few who are entrusted with a patient's care, to make a direct difference in people's lives and well-being, to deliver a newborn into the world, or to hold the hand of the dying.

Do not take this charge lightly.

No matter how dull the case, no matter how annoying the patient, be humble in your role. Respect the responsibility you carry. And, above all else, respect your patients. Be dedicated to them, and let them continue to teach you for all your years of practice. Strive to achieve that elusive balance in your personal and professional lives so that you can truly serve those you care for and those who care for you.

Finally, as someone who has run the gauntlet and survived the medical training process, consider the opportunity to give back. Look around, and you will find many young faces not unlike yours a number of years ago, eager, confused, and afraid. Take the time to be a mentor, to offer advice and counsel. Above all, offer the encouragement that can lead young students to have confidence in themselves. We stand together as physicians in no small part because of the diligent efforts and unending encouragement of those who came before us.

Long may the tradition continue.

PART SEVEN

Advice for the
Spouses, Partners,
Significant Others,
and Families of
Med Students

CHAPTER 29

The Realities of Life with a Doc-in-Training and Strategies for Making It Livable

by Kimberly Bissell

Life is like a diaper . . . short and loaded.
—PROVERB

SURE," I SAID, "go to medical school."

What was it to me, really? We were dating, and while I liked him a lot there was little chance we'd settle down together, right?

Well, here I am, writing a chapter about what it's like to be married to a medical student. His training has shaped our lives and our children's lives for the last ten years. We started dating when he applied and got married in his second year of med school. We had our first child during his third year and our second child in the middle of his residency. We've moved once for residency and again for a job. Our story is hardly unique. Now, *your* significant other or family member is considering medical school. While the focus of this chapter is about what it's like to marry a med student, much of the information and coping techniques apply to close family and friends as well.

If your significant other is contemplating donning the stethoscope and you're reading this chapter, you're probably not married yet or only newly married. If you don't already have children, you'll likely want to have them eventually. You're probably going to school or working full-time yourself. And mostly . . . you're not sure how to feel about your significant other becoming a doctor.

You're not alone.

This chapter is intended to help educate you about what to expect, both good and bad, from your med student and their schedule. I'll present some expectations you should have for him or her as well as what they're going to need from you during this process. And finally, I'll provide some coping strategies for surviving the tough times and enjoying the good ones.

Most important, know this: your relationship can survive medical school. You may even grow together through the experience. Ultimately your success or failure will depend on the balance you strike with each other in your relationship and the balance you achieve as individuals with separate interests. Together you can meet the challenges medical school presents, but it's going to take a lot of open communication and patience from both of you.

WHY SHOULD I WORRY?

Two realizations pop up right off the bat when you first learn of your partner's interest in becoming a doctor: "Cool, we'll be able to afford a house and nice cars someday," and, "Come on, is it *really* that hard to go to medical school?"

It's no myth that doctors have good salaries. As a whole, they're not making what they used to make (at least that's what everyone tells you), but you will be able to support your family comfortably on your spouse's income. The aging population and ongoing health-care crisis mean physicians are likely to remain in high demand. In all likelihood, your spouse will have a good chance at finding a job. Depending on the competitiveness of their chosen specialty, you may have to move for residency and/or for the first job, but opportunities are out there.

What you will discover is that it *really is* that hard to go to medical school. It's damn near impossible to get into and it completely takes over your life when you do. Your spouse will be breathing, eating, and sleeping medicine for the next seven to ten years. And even after residency is over, chances are they'll be so attuned to breathing, eating, and sleeping medicine they'll require a certain amount of retraining. Unfortunately, your life will require a certain amount of breathing and eating medicine as well. The realities of marrying a med student will affect where you live, how you live, and the sacrifices you'll have to make along the way.

THE TOP FIVE REALITIES ABOUT MARRYING A MED STUDENT

1. **They study and work long hours.** Your partner or significant other *will* work really long hours. Unfortunately, even with new restrictions in residency programs, they will still work insane hours and have little time to think of anything or anyone else. The good part is that hard months are often coupled with easy months, and you will find they do have free time during the year to catch up on being a human.

2. **They will receive little or no salary for a long time.** Envision four years of expensive schooling (medical-school tuition is one of the highest in graduate education) followed by three to five years of little pay. You have to be prepared for the long haul of cheap living and loan stress. In addition, while you're rebelling against the thought of another box of mac and cheese, many of your friends who are dating or are married to lawyers, investment bankers, entrepreneurs, or other professionals will be living the high life. You will realize the opportunity cost of years of low or no salary from your spouse. Have that box of mac and cheese and carefully consider what you can reasonably afford in your life. The less debt you incur in loans or credit cards, the more freedom you will have down the road, especially when it comes to choosing a specialty.

3. **They have little control over their time.** Your partner signed up to become a doctor with the understanding that there would be lifestyle sacrifices. What most soon-to-be med students don't always think about is the sacrifice that their family, friends, and spouses also have to make, even if they're not married yet. Once those applications and match lists are sent out, any one of the locations applied to could be your new home. An acceptance letter from a school in a faraway city is a hard thing to turn down after years of premed toil and stress.

4. **They have a hard time finding a balance.** It will seem that there is an endless stream of information that your spouse has to know. It's not possible for them to learn it all and still have huge blocks of free time every day. Most of the time they'll be studying or working in the hospital. On occasion, it will be hard for them to even break for lunch. There will always be more work to be done.

5. **Your own life and career will be marginalized.** It can be difficult to compete when your spouse is late because a grieving family needed attention or a woman went into labor. It can be impossible to still think your needs are important and very hard for your partner to calm down and concentrate on home life.

"Whew," you're saying to yourself. "Life isn't supposed to be this hard! Will it really be that awful for the next ten years?"

The answer is no. The pains and joys of med school ebb and flow like anything else. Much will depend on how you work out your day-to-day life, plan your fun, and compromise on the small stuff. The bottom line is that you should invest yourself in understanding what med school is all about as it will affect your life, too.

How Will Your Med Student Be Spending His or Her Time?

The medical training process is long and very confusing to outsiders. Each phase has distinct advantages and challenges for couples and families. Here's a thumbnail sketch of the phases and what you can expect from each.

Applying to school/premed years

Applying to medical school is one of the two most stressful times during the tenure of medical training. (The other will be preparing for Match Day for residency.) Not only will your partner be spending thousands of dollars and years of time preparing to take the MCATs, struggling to excel in prerequisite classes, and completing all of the inane paperwork and applications only to wait impatiently for a response, they will also be second-guessing choices at every turn. Even if your partner is incredibly self-assured, it will become your job to help sort through conflicting emotions about going to medical school at some point during this process. This can be a very precarious position as you want to be supportive, but at the same time this may not feel like the right choice for *you*. You've probably been able to keep yourself at a distance from the "future life" discussions up until now, and you're just beginning to realize that this is life-altering stuff going on.

Engage in these discussions with your future med student and become a team player. The decision of where to apply will directly affect you as well.

Once your med student has been accepted and has made the decision to go, try to decide *where* together. Chances are good that you may have to leave your job, family, or close friends to make a new life in another city. Look at jobs in your new market, check housing costs, think about your interests, and determine which of your location choices might have the most opportunity for you to do things that you like. It will be disillusioning to arrive in a new city only to realize that you are spending a great deal of time alone or with a gaggle of medical students. The faster you can find avenues for your interests, the less resentful you'll be of your partner and his new life.

Preclinical training (or the first few years of med school)

That first couple of years of school seem blissful to me now, although at the time I found them to be a stressful transition from both of us working. You will start to feel the pull of your new role in logistical and emotional support for your partner's newfound life. The best news is that while your spouse will have a ton of classes and labs, plus work to prepare and memorize, evenings and weekends are open. Granted, a majority of that time will be dedicated to studying, but most important, med students will have the freedom to schedule out-of-school time. You may even be able to block off regular time together every day. Your joint time will be more constrained, however, as they will feel the constant pull of the books.

In addition, your med-student partner will have regularly scheduled school breaks and the first summer off. Watching your med student relax back into the person you once knew and loved is very reassuring, even if short-lived. Take advantage of these early vacations. Spend as much time together as possible. Vacation cheaply and do all major house projects or moves during these times.

Clinical training in med school

At the end of the second year of school, most med schools start sending their students on clinical rotations. The daily routine is no longer at the discretion of your med student, and the pressure of treating actual patients and answering to actual physicians rises.

Many rotations will include call nights where med students usually sleep at the hospital—if they sleep at all—and return home the following day around noon. Then they'll crash and sleep through the afternoon and night, only to have to be back at the hospital the next morning. When they're not at the hospital, they will still be expected to read and prepare for end-of-rotation tests or papers. Most rotations will last about a month, and with every change there will be a whole new crew of coworkers to meet and systems to learn. Some months will be blissful, with an easy schedule—no call and hopefully a subject your partner loves. Others will be sheer hell.

Be prepared for a change in attitude from your partner once clinical rotations begin. They'll be much happier, even though working hours increase. Clinical training is exhilarating to most med students—after all, treating patients is why they went to med school. Unfortunately, it also signals the end of their day-to-day freedom. They always have to show up and rarely get to make their own schedules. For those of you working in the real world, this may be a welcome change as most months they'll have a 7 A.M. to 6 P.M. working schedule, have time during the day to study, and will be truly free some evenings and weekends.

Some of the worst rotations in terms of schedule are surgery, medicine, ob/gyn, and emergency medicine. During these months, they will get the least amount of sleep because the hours are odd or early and there will be regular call shifts where they are responsible for a number of patients through the night. They'll come home exhausted and demoralized. All day long, everyone will have been asking them questions about what they know in the particular specialty, and they will be required to perform on almost no sleep. It's as bad as you've seen on any TV show. Do not plan to get married, have a baby, or go on an expensive vacation during these critical, stressful rotations. You will be disappointed at your partner's ability to help out or actively participate in something that is so important to you and should be to both of you.

By the fourth year, things will start moving hard and fast. During the year your med student will be choosing a specialty, applying to residency, and interviewing around the country. The range of diverse specialties offer varying lifestyles in the long run, and depending on the aspirations of your partner, your life could look very different if you are married to a cardiovascular surgeon or a family practitioner. Again, just like the med-school decision, be engaged in the choices and vocal about your hopes and needs for you and your future or current family. If possible, you should travel with your partner to the matching interviews at the most interesting programs. It helps keep at bay the intense feelings that you lack all control in the process.

A word of warning: there is a ton of gossip and hearsay about programs and specialties, both within med-school circles and on the interview trail. You will feel unsure of how your partner stands at any program until the end. By Match Day, you will feel totally overwhelmed and completely freaked out.

Hang in there.

By the last spring of med school, after Match Day and before residency, your partner will feel more comfortable on the wards and will be excited about medicine, about you, and about the world. During their fourth year, most med students self-schedule their blocks of rotations and, yes, *vacations!* Many students try to pack their hard rotations at the beginning of the year to help weight their application for residency, and push their easy or free months until the end. In fact, Dan had almost three months off at the end of school. It was a blissful break. This is a great time to plan big life events, including a move. A lot of our friends either planned weddings or had babies near the end of fourth year in order to enjoy some kind of family leave. Be sure to take time off together. Try to leave medicine behind for a while.

Internship and residency

At last, they're working, and hopefully in a field that they're excited about.

At this stage of our experience, I remember thinking that Dan and I could handle anything, now that he had finished med school and we had moved across the country. In a way, I was right. We'd established our systems for coping through incredibly hard months. The problem with internship and residency is that you find yourself coping for much longer periods of time. The easier months come fewer and farther between, and sleep deprivation becomes a part of your daily life. During these years, your med student has an overwhelming sense of responsibility to the hospital that seems unending.

These will be the times when you will wonder what you have gotten yourself into by falling in love with a doctor, especially if you have children. Keep reminding yourself that life *will* get better. Remind yourself regularly that many other couples have successfully charted this course before you.

HOW TO SURVIVE MED SCHOOL
AS A SPOUSE, PARTNER, OR SIGNIFICANT OTHER

Before you start this long road your med student needs to know and understand a few things:

1. You are not going to medical school, but you *do* have another life that isn't all about medical school. This isn't your career choice, but it significantly impacts you.
2. You and your partner are a pair—you also need life support, both logistically and emotionally.
3. Your partner will need to listen to your feelings about school choices and be willing to make compromises. Like it or not, this career is about you, too.
4. You will be making serious sacrifices and your partner needs to be appreciative.

It's important that you remember to protect your interests, livelihood, and identity, even when you feel swept up in those of your spouse. Nevertheless, be prepared to provide a lot, including:

- **Emotional support.** One of the hardest things about med school is getting accepted. When med students start school they feel like everyone else is smarter and more prepared than they are. This is normal. Try to make your med student feel like success in medical school is possible. They will need the opportunity to whine about the workload, the lack of enthusiasm, the long hours, and the tough patients. At times, all you'll ever hear about is how hard med school is for your partner, despite the fact that you will feel like med school is pretty damned hard for you, too.
- **Financial and household support.** While it might seem important to have your partner evenly share household tasks and financial contribution, it's not realistic to believe that will hap-

pen. Try to see your life as a long-term partnership, and your investment will pay off as your med student chips in with home-cooked meals and a clean house during easy rotations, and vacations and financial security in the future. Use the free time on breaks to accomplish major house projects or cleaning sessions, and try not to fill your short time together arguing about who last cleaned the floor.

- **Flexibility.** Your med student will be late and/or exhausted during many social engagements you share. The last-minute study/lab sessions, rotation or scheduling changes, and staying late on a shift or on a postcall morning will be regular occurrences. Try to be clear about what major calendar events are crucial and be flexible about everything else. Again, if you're not flexible, you'll spend hours arguing about things you can't change.

- **Patience and understanding.** The classic story is the spouse who is angry and abusive when his or her med student comes home late from a shift only to learn that the med student's last hour was spent with a family who'd lost a loved one. Before jumping to conclusions, try to hear the explanation and keep in mind how little sleep and how much pressure your med student is getting.

- **No guilt trips.** Making your med student feel guilty about how little you feel supported will only make you both feel bad. Similarly, however, don't let yourself feel guilty for getting out with your friends or continuing to do things that you love to do, even if your partner can't join you. You'll feel less resentment and be able to be more patient and understanding about what your med student is going through. All in all, the more balance you create in your own life, the happier you'll be and the more your partner will want to come home and join you.

- **Gentle reminders about balance.** Be the gentle reminder that your med student needs to rest, eat well, exercise, and stay mentally healthy. It's important to not get caught up in the pressure of school and performance on the wards. Med students will be more successful if they get out of the hospital more frequently than they think they can. If that means bringing dinner to the hospital on a call night or letting your med student sleep in at home when possible, do it.

- **Downtime alone.** The one thing that I frequently forget about Dan is that he gets very little downtime alone. Most of his hobbies or interests fell to the wayside when med school began and we got married. When he's home, I always have a list of things we need to accomplish or friends and family we should see. I have to remind myself that he needs time to himself to recharge.

While it may seem that your partner's needs are unending and your nerves are regularly frayed, things will usually get better. This is a long road and medical school is only the first part of the training. Most of your coping skills will be put to the test during your partner's internship year. We've already touched upon some of the coping strategies listed below. Use this expanded list as a reference during stressful times. Hang in there and know that you're not alone.

COPING TIPS

- **Keep living your life.** Just because your significant other can't hang out with friends and family doesn't mean you can't. Be sure to still enjoy the activities that you love even if you must enjoy them alone. It will be hard for both of you, but you will resent your partner less if you don't spend hours waiting to do something together.
- **Find a social and emotional support system.** If you've moved to a new city, be sure to find a way to meet people and make friends. It's lonely when you're on your third weekend alone in the month and it seems like everyone else is out with their boyfriend or girlfriend. Many med schools have spouses' groups that get together every so often. Make friends with other spouses—they know what you're experiencing better than anyone and can often make suggestions about ways to cope, or they can just provide emotional support. During med school and residency, a bunch of us started getting together regularly for dinner. Most of us were new to the area and we quickly became fast friends.
- **Get rid of the guilt.** Try not to make your med student feel guilty for things they already feel bad about, and try not to let them make you feel guilty because you're not in med school. Set reasonable expectations and then be very frank when your med student isn't meeting them. Give them time to make things up to you.

- **Be clear about your needs and boundaries.** Med school will take over both of your lives if you're not careful. Decide early on what you need from the relationship for it to survive, then set clear boundaries on what does and doesn't work for you. Again, these expectations have to be reasonable or you'll fight over them all the time. I really needed a little one-on-one time with my husband every week—no TV, no kids, no parents, no friends, just the two of us and some time to catch up when he wasn't asleep. I also hated waiting for us both to clean the house, so we stretched a corner of the budget and found a way to pay someone to do it for us. If you're clear about what your basic needs are, your partner can do everything possible to meet them and can make it up to you when it's not. Sometimes it will not be enough, but it will help you survive the rough months.

- **Have opinions and express them gently.** Try to listen to your med student's trials and tribulations, ask a lot of questions, and take an active part in decision making about a medical career. Most choices will affect both your lives. Play an active role in discussions about your med student's specialty choice and talk about the residency programs of interest. Do research on your own about which cities to live in and which programs encourage resident wellness. Be a sounding board but don't be afraid to formulate and express your own opinions about what might be best for you as a couple.

- **Don't hide your emotions.** Being afraid to tell your med student that you are unhappy will only create resentment that you can't shake. Speak up when you were hoping for different outcomes and when you're happy that things are working out. Time wasted on wondering how the other is feeling is time you could have spent doing something fun together. Talk about what you're thinking about and try to let it go. Med students don't have extra time for worry.

- **Combine your calendars.** It's stressful to you when your med student disregards important, planned events, and it's stressful to him when you've planned them during major study pushes or hard rotations. Try to understand what months and which classes will be overwhelming and be respectful. At the same time, get important dates like weddings on the calendar so your med student can get those days off early and won't agree to volunteer at the homeless clinic in the middle of that weekend.

IS THE END EVER IN SIGHT?

Truthfully, yes and no. Residency will be much worse in terms of sleep deprivation and free time at home. But your doctor partner will have more responsibility, more control, and will be hassled less by the attending physicians. They'll be happier. They also can start looking at their work as work, and therefore leave it behind them at the end of the shift. Depending on the specialty that your spouse chooses, medicine may always be a lot of hours and focus in their life. Being that so many docs start out hoping to "help people," that's usually what we love most about them. The best advice we ever received is to help your spouse and yourself keep some balance in your life. Everyone does their job better when they are able to step away from it once in a while.

You can survive medical school as a spouse. All it takes is a lot of patience, care, and understanding about your and your partner's mutual needs. Because the training is so thorough and the workload is so intense, becoming a doctor is not a decision to make lightly. In the end, the benefit to being a life partner to a doctor is knowing that your partner really is helping people feel better, and you can find solace in the knowledge that in no small way, you helped to make that happen.

Appendix

M EDICINE IS AN inherently dynamic field—thus the information sources are eternally changing and growing. This appendix lists some of the most fundamental resources premed students, med students, and residents will draw on during their journey. But the list is only the tip of that ever-changing iceberg. Talk to your fellow students, talk to your colleagues, faculty, and mentors, and you will discover a world of resources available to you.

We would be remiss if we did not also add a note of warning. As you well know, the Internet is awesome in its breadth and variety, but sometimes questionable in its quality. Before you depend on a resource make sure that is it is reputable and has up-to-date material. Furthermore, medicine is big business, and medical training is in and of itself a major industry. There are many companies out there trying to sell you the one resource you can't do without. You will discover that in your mild paranoia and desire to succeed, you can spend a small fortune on references and materials only to be eternally burdened by a library you never get around to reading or a resource that tells you what you already know. Be a cautious consumer and consider who's offering the advice before you take it. To this end, it should be noted that the authors have no association with any vendors, organizations, or individuals listed here, nor can we vouch for the ever-changing content of these resources. Nonetheless, many, many students have found these links and resources useful in their journey, and we hope that they will offer at least a starting point for your exploration into the world ahead of you.

FUNDAMENTAL REFERENCES

These Web sites offer comprehensive information on the medical training experience from stem to stern. They should be among your go-to resources throughout your journey for up-to-date, high-quality information and guidance.

- **Association of American Medical Colleges** (www.aamc.org): This should *always* be your first stop when shopping for *any* information regarding the premedical, medical, or postgraduate training and experience. The breadth and depth of this Web site is awesome. Even though it is directed more specifically at allopathic training, osteopaths will find much of its content extremely useful as well.
- **American Association of Colleges of Osteopathic Medicine** (www.aacom.org): This is the osteopathic version of the AAMC Web site. It, too, contains a fantastic array of information, resources, and links. Make it your launching point for any osteopathic investigations.
- **Student Doctor Network** (www.studentdoctor.net): SDN is a nonprofit organization that started as a grassroots Web community at the University of Kansas in the mid-1990s. Since then it has emerged as one of the most comprehensive and most useful student-driven resources out there. Perhaps its strongest feature is the incredible "Student Doctor Forums." These e-mail forums detail literally every aspect of the premed and medical student experience and provide a real-time community to raise questions, vent frustrations, and learn from the collective wisdom of those around you and before you.

TEST PREP

There's a wide range of MCAT prep courses and books out there. These resources change all the time, so talk to your colleagues and advisors about what they feel are the best options currently. For test prep courses, Kaplan and Princeton Review remain the heavy hitters. Their courses may not be perfect, but they do put you through the paces, enforce proactive studying, and offer full-length simulated tests to get you ready for the big day. For specifics about registration and test content, go to the governing organizations directly and download their materials.

- The Princeton Review: www.princetonreview.com
- Kaplan: www.kaplan.com
- MCAT home page: www.aamc.org/students/mcat/start.htm
- USMLE home page: www.usmle.org
- COMLEX home page: www.nbome.org

PREMED CURRICULUM AND MED-SCHOOL APPLICATIONS

Your premed advisor is your best initial source of premed information. They typically will have a library of reference materials and a wealth of experience in guiding you through the process. Additional resources are listed below.

- The AAMC Web site (www.aamc.org) is probably the best single premed resource. They publish the official tome *Medical School Admission Requirements,* which is widely regarded as the bible on facts about medical schools and what it takes to gain acceptance to one. Again, your premed advisor may have a copy of this book, so look before you invest. The AAMC Web site also lists every premed program available in the country.
- Online you will find a wide variety of course synopses and study materials for all the different premed classes. Again, quality may vary, so consider who's offering the information before you rely on it. Amazon.com is a good first stop for these materials.
- The Student Doctor Network (www.studentdoctor.net) has extensive reviews of online material and entire forums that discuss each course you'll have to take. Learn from the legions that have gone into premed battle before you.

CLINICAL REFERENCES

By the time you're enrolled in med-school classes, you'll have an entire cadre of fellow students clamoring to find the best study resources available. Use the collective wisdom of those who have gone before you. Try out any reference before you invest a lot of money in it—some books and materials may suit your learning style better than others. When in doubt, buy fewer rather than more general reference books. Your best bet, by and large, will be high-yield, topic-specific review books that will help focus your studies on the most pertinent material for tests and clinics. Remember to gradually and continuously study for the upcoming USMLE tests as you go—you'll thank yourself later. Here are some of the classics, always a good place to start.

Web Sites

There are a number of excellent online reference sources that provide ubiquitous access and up-to-date materials. Your medical school likely has subscriptions to these services already through its library. If not, you may want to consider subscribing yourself—the information can be so high-yield that it can save you literally hours of searching at critical times.

- **UpToDate** (www.uptodate.com). While generally focused on internal medicine, this site contains succinct reviews of current thinking and treatment about most major disease processes. Their articles are only a couple of pages long and are generally authored by leaders in the field. They include bibliographies for each entry, substantiating their recommendations and making further research a breeze. This should be your first stop at 2 A.M. over a cup of coffee as you begin to write up your fourth admission H & P for the night.
- **MD Consult** (www.mdconsult.com). This site is literally an entire library at your fingertips. They provide a wide array of the major textbooks for most medical specialities in an online searchable format. The material is dense (i.e., it's straight from the textbook), but its searchable format allows you to hone in on specific information quickly.
- **Micromedex** (www.micromedex.com). This site is best known for its comprehensive database of drugs and toxins. It provides concise, current information on thousands of compounds and their impact on humans—both therapeutic and toxic. Micromedex also offers a range of other products, including differential diagnosis utilities, treatment guidelines, and patient-education databases.

- **eMedicine** (www.emedicine.com). This site is similar to UpTo-Date but offers a wider range of subspecialty topics. It, too, prides itself on keeping its content current by recruiting its authors from a wide range of experts in the field and conducting regular reviews of its articles.
- *The Merck Manual of Diagnosis and Therapy* (www.merck.com/mrkshared/mmanual/home.jsp). First published in 1899, this book has remained a solid general medical reference for medical practitioners around the world. The online version is easily searchable and quite succinct.

PDA Resources

PDAs have emerged as a more efficient and less weighty means of carrying an entire library in your white-coat pocket. Many schools now require or provide them as part of the curriculum. Again, there are a wealth of products out there, some good, some not so good. Here are a couple of the most tried-and-true, as well as some good clearing houses for more products and information.

- **Epocrates** (www2.epocrates.com). This is probably the single best freeware drug reference for the PDA. There are certainly others to pick from, but most require a subscription of some sort and offer relatively little more for your money. Epocrates also offers additional subscriber-only functions, such as Infectious Disease references, if you feel the need.
- **Griffith's 5-Minute Clinical Consult** (www.5mcc.com). You will encounter countless moments in your medical training when you find yourself in the elevator on the way down to the ER to admit a patient with Kawasaki's disease, and you think to yourself, "Uh oh, what the heck do I remember about Kawasaki's disease?" Witness Griffith's five-minute clinical consult to the rescue. It's concise, it's easy to navigate, and it consistently hits the high points you need to know before you walk into the exam room or sit down to write orders on a patient. It won't replace reading a good review article or textbook to really learn about a disease process, but it can easily serve to jog your memory and get you out of a pinch in a hurry.
- **Medical PDA Software.** There is a wide range of Web sites dedicated to medical software for your PDA. There are huge volumes of freeware, some if which is high-quality and extremely

useful, some of which is liable to crash your system or provide faulty information. There are also numerous commercial products that all claim to be the one, indispensable PDA resource. Remember that there's no information panacea out there—in the end, you've got to know what you need to know. These PDA programs will serve as excellent quick-reference tools and calculators, but don't be fooled into thinking they'll solve any problems for you. Used judiciously to fill information gaps, your PDA will be your best assistant. If you load it with extraneous programs and reams of data in hopes of never being caught off guard for a pimping session, you'll quickly find you've wasted money and time when you should have been paying attention to patients and learning what you need to know.

Pocket Reference Library

Let's face it, sometimes nothing beats flipping through the pages of a well-worn, trusted book to find that drug dose immediately. Plus, you never have to worry about crashes or battery life. Here are a couple of classic, all-around pocket reference books, most of which should be available through your school's bookstore.

- *Sanford Guide* (www.sanfordguide.com). This is probably the preeminent guide to antimicrobial therapy. It's dense and in very fine print, but ultimately you will find exactly the right bug-to-drug combination if you spend some time scrutinizing it.
- Tarascon (www.tarascon.com). This company is most renowned for its pharmacopoeia, but it also produces a range of specialty-specific quick-reference books. When your PDA crashes and you need to know the dose, here's a quick and cheap backup.
- *Practical Guide to the Care of the Medical Patient,* edited by Fred F. Ferri (Mosby); *The Washington Manual of Medical Therapeutics* (Lippincott, Williams, and Wilkins); *The Harriet Lane Handbook* [Mosby]. These three books are among the most popular of the generic hard-copy clinical pocket reference books. To the third- and fourth-year student embroiled in a clinical rotation, they can be indispensable sources of information on what needs to be in an admission order set, the exact steps to put in a subclavian central line, or how to safely rehydrate a child with IV fluids. There are many similar books out there, but these have stood the test of time and developed a legendary status

among generations of students. Find one that suits your thinking and have it at the ready in your bag.

FINANCES

As we mentioned in chapter 11, there is a wide range of funding sources available to make it feasible for almost anyone to undertake a medical education. The key is sorting through your options and crafting the best financial-aid package. Start by looking for scholarships and grants, then move to on to federal loans and private loans. You may be surprised by the scholarship and grant monies you discover if you hunt around. Remember, even a relatively small $10,000 grant from a local civic organization can save you tens of thousands of dollars over the thirty-year time frame of your loan package repayment. Here are a few places to start, but search the Internet, talk to your school, and reach out to your community to see what you can find.

- **Federal Student Aid** (www.studentaid.ed.gov). This is the place to start for any federal support. You will have to fill out the Free Application for Federal Student Aid in order to get a needs evaluation and package proposal. Your financial-aid advisor can help you navigate these waters, but this Web site will also give you reams of information on how to apply for loans and how to manage your loans come repayment time.
- **Scholarship Resources.** There are a number of scholarship clearing houses on the Internet that will allow you to access their databases for a fee. This may be worth your while, but it's probably best to first check with your financial-aid advisor on resources they already have available. Again, don't forget to investigate your hometown resources, particularly civic organizations, churches, and schools.
- **Service Repayment Options.** Want to wipe out your loan debt completely and serve your country at the same time? Consider a stint in the National Health Service Corps (http://nhsc.bhpr .hrsa.gov) in exchange for a partial or complete loan repayment. Or you might wish to join a branch of the armed services. They will help support you while you're in school, assist with residency placement, and repay your student loans in ex-

change for several years of active-duty service. The commitments to any of these programs are significant and may change your life, but then again so will being debt free.

RESIDENCY AND THE MATCH

By now you will have a deep working knowledge of the medical education system as well as an entire Student Affairs office at your school assisting you with entering and competing in the match. Use these resources well, and ask many, many questions. Here are a few additional sites you may want to consider.

- **FREIDA Online** (www.ama-assn.org/ama/pub/category/2997 .html). This portion of the AMA Web site is dedicated to a fantastic database on all the available fields of training. They not only provide useful statistics on the field and the lifestyle, they also provide links to all the approved residencies in that field. This is a great place to start shopping around and exploring your interests.
- **Electronic Residency Application Service (ERAS)** (www.aamc .org/students/eras/start.htm). Yet another part of the monolithic AAMC Web site, ERAS is your gateway to residency acceptance. The system is analogous to your medical-school applications, with the exception of those miserable secondary applications. Early in the application process (i.e., before it truly begins), spend some time on this Web site learning about the ERAS application, the system for submission and interviews, and most important, the deadlines and requirements. Don't let inattention to detail allow you to miss a critical step or deadline and derail this most important, life-changing process.
- **National Resident Matching Program** (www.nrmp.org). This is the counterpart to the ERAS application. The NRMP are the folks who will take your rank list, crunch you and the thousands of other applicants through a wickedly complex algorithm, and single-handedly determine your future. Again, early on in the process you should scrutinize this site and make sure you understand the system and what you need to do to successfully complete the requirements.

RESOURCES FOR FAMILY, FRIENDS, AND SUPPORTERS

As we discussed in part seven, the stress and strain of medical training affect not just you but also those closest to you. Here are a few Web sites dedicated to creating a network of support for those you rely on. No one can dissolve the stress and strain, but sometimes a voice of solidarity and experience can ease the burden and offer guidance.

- **AMA Alliance** (www.ama-assn.org/ama/pub/category/2109 .html). This is by far the oldest organization dedicated to addressing the well-being of physicians and their families. The original "Women's Auxiliary to the AMA" was started in 1922. Since then the organization has grown to encompass all physician families in any stage of training from medical school to retirement. They offer regional chapters, publications, guidance, and opportunities to get involved in health policy. It's definitely worth checking out, and it may help your significant other feel like he can be a more active part of the medical training process.
- **MomMD** (www.mommd.com). While this site is dedicated to the issues of women in medicine and the unique challenges they face, it offers a wealth of information about how to achieve balance in your life, no matter your gender or living situation. It offers extensive tips and resources for every stage of training invaluable to both would-be physicians and their families.

ABOUT THE AUTHORS

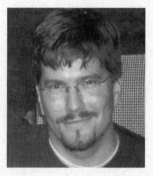

ROBERT MILLER graduated with distinction from Yale University in 1993 and from the University of Pennsylvania Law School, where he served as a senior editor of the *Law Review* and chairman of the Executive Committee on Student Ethics and Academic Standing, in 1998. He is presently a trial lawyer at Sheehan, Phinney, Bass & Green in Manchester, New Hampshire, where he specializes in constitutional law and intellectual-property issues. He is the author of *Law School Confidential, Business School Confidential,* and *Campus Confidential.* Mr. Miller lives in Hopkinton, New Hampshire, with his wife, Carolyn, and their two children.

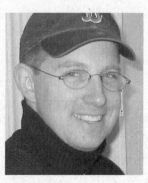

DR. DAN BISSELL graduated from the University of Colorado School of Medicine in 2002. He recently completed his residency in emergency medicine at the Maine Medical Center. During residency he received the Gold Foundation Award as Resident Teacher of the Year and was appointed chief resident of the emergency medicine program.

Prior to his medical training, Dan was involved in a number of pursuits. He graduated cum laude from Middlebury College in 1993 with a major in geology. He spent two years conducting marine geophysical research, much of it spent at sea mapping the ocean floor. Back on land he entered the computer mapping industry, working for utility and environmental clients. He went on to cofound Jupiter Technologies, a GIS and custom software engineering firm. He completed his premed studies at the University of Colorado while running the business.

Dr. Bissell lives (and practices) in Portland, Oregon, with his wife, Kim, and their two children. Kim authored the final section on surviving as a spouse in the medical world.